Southwest Scientific Publishing
P.O. Box 10
Dalhart, TX 79022
U.S.A.

The intelligent person's alternative to
fad diets and health/nutrition misinformation.

THIRD—CLASS MAIL
US POSTAGE
PAID
Dalhart, TX 79022
Permit No. 106

Our motto:

Scientific Accuracy

with maximum

Readability

INTELLIGENT

DIETING

for
Weight Loss
and
Prevention of Disease

D. PORTER PRICE Ph.D.

Published and Distributed by
SOUTHWEST SCIENTIFIC
P. O. Box 10
Dalhart, Texas 79022
United States of America

Telephone 806-249-4727

ISBN 0-9606246-1-9 Hardcover
ISBN 0-9606246-2-7 Softcover

Typesetting by
Loftin Printing

TABLE OF CONTENTS

CHAPTER 1   PREFACE/INTRODUCTION AND   1
THE DANGER IN HEALTH FOOD FADS AND CRASH DIETS

SECTION I — DIET AND WEIGHT LOSS   **8**

CHAPTER 2   UNDERSTANDING HUNGER   9
(WHY WE BECOME AS HUNGRY OR HUNGRIER WHEN
WE DO OFFICEWORK AS WHEN WE DO PHYSICAL WORK)
  Hunger Mechanisms   9
  Skipping a Meal   11
  Nutritional Considerations   12
  Summary   12

CHAPTER 3   WHY CALORIE COUNTING CAN BE   13
MISLEADING

CHAPTER 4   DIETING TO MAKE US MORE ATTRACTIVE   19
RATHER THAN JUST THIN

CHAPTER 5   THE REVOLUTIONARY UNBALANCED DIET   22

CHAPTER 6   AN EFFECTIVE DIET PLAN   26
  Basic Premise   27
  First Step   27
  Second Step   32
  Third Step — Losing Weight   33
  Educated Meal Planning   34
  Dieting Tips   40
  Types of Sugar   42
  Putting It All Together   43

CHAPTER 7   VITAMINS AND MINERALS   46
(WHAT WE NEED AND DON'T NEED)
  The Recommended Daily Allowances (RDAs)   50
  Notes on Sample Diet   50
  Conclusions   54

CHAPTER 8   EXERCISE — AN INTEGRAL PART OF   57
ANY DIET/HEALTH PLAN
  Effect Upon the Heart   59
  Physiological Differences in Exercises   59
  How to Begin an Exercise Program   61

Selecting and Beginning a Basic Program 62
Individual Exercise Programs 63
Summary and Final Thoughts 63

CHAPTER 9   ALCOHOL IN THE DIET 65
Calories Added to the Diet 65
Changes in the Digestive Tract 66
Summary and Conclusions 67

SECTION II — DIET, NUTRITION, AND HEALTH 68

CHAPTER 10   NUTRITION AND RESISTANCE TO 69
INFECTIOUS DISEASES
Infectious Agents 69
Antibiotics 69
Controlling Viral Diseases 70
Factors Affecting the Ability to Produce Antibodies 72
Fighting Colds, Flu, and Other Viral Diseases 72
Interferon 73
Summary 75

CHAPTER 11   DIET AND HYPERACTIVITY IN CHILDREN 76
The Condition 76
The Food Additive Free Diet 76
Scientific Evaluation 77
Opinion of Physicians and Scientists 77
Other Theories 78
Megavitamin Treatment 78
Sugar 78
Common Sense Conclusions (Author's Opinion) 78

CHAPTER 12   DIET AND DIABETES 83
Physiological Problems Faced by Diabetics 84
Diets for Diabetics 85
Diet in the Prevention of Diabetes 86

CHAPTER 13   HYPERTENSION (HIGH BLODD PRESSURE) 88
Primary Hypertension 88
Cutting Down on Salt 91
Special Needs 91

CHAPTER 14   NUTRITIONAL ASPECTS OF HEART DISEASE 94
The Cholesterol Controversy 94
Atherosclerosis 94

The Compound 97
Early Research 98
Later Research with Laboratory Animals 98
Cholesterol Metabolism in Man 98
Recent Research 99
High Blood Cholesterol 99
Dietary Recommendations for Hypercholesterolemia 101
Dietary Recommendations for Normal People 101
Other Dietary Factors 102
Sugar 102
Alcohol 106
Cigarette Smoking 107
Conclusions on Heart Disease and Diet 108

CHAPTER 15   DIET, NUTRITION, AND CANCER 113
Naturally Occurring Carcinogens in the Food Supply 113
Nutritional Aspects of Hormonally Induced Cancers 119
Food Additives and Cancer 123
Pesticides 125
Drugs Used in Livestock 126
Intentional Additives 127
Tobacco and Alcohol 128
Summary of the Nutritional Aspects of Cancer 130

CHAPTER 16   DIVERTICULITIS (INFLAMED BOWEL) 132

SECTION III — REFERENCE 133

CHAPTER 17   LOW CALORIE COOKING 134
Dessert Toppings 136
Gelatin 137
Use of Yogurt, Cottage Cheese, or Sour Cream 137
Whole Wheat Flour 138
Foods Other Than Desserts and Pastries 139
Summary 140

CHAPTER 18   VITAMINS 141

CHAPTER 19   MINERALS 159
Macro-Minerals 159
Trace Minerals 162

CHAPTER 20   BASIC DIGESTION AND METABOLISM 170

Anatomy and Physiology of Digestion   170
Utilization of Carbohydrate   172
Protein Metabolism   173
Digestion and Utilization of Fats   176
Types of Fats   176
Summary   177

LITERATURE CITED   178

GLOSSARY   181

INDEX   185

Chapter 1 PREFACE/INTRODUCTION
AND
THE DANGER IN HEALTH FOOD FADS AND CRASH DIETS

As U.S. Citizens we enjoy freedoms unprecedented in the rest of the world. One of those precious freedoms we enjoy is the freedom of speech. Designed to protect us from an oppressive political regime, the First Ammendment was written to provide each political faction the right to express its views. Without freedom of speech, a democracy cannot exist.

While the overall value of freedom of speech has to be overwhelmingly positive, there are negative aspects. The negative aspects come in the form of misinformation. In the area of diet and health, there is an enormous amount of misinformation available to the public.

This misinformation is promulgated by two different methods and motivations:

1. Well intentioned but ill advised people, who sincerely believe that what they are saying is true.
2. Unscrupulous individuals hoping to merchandise a product through the use of fraudulent claims and/or scientific inaccuracies and half-truths. Unfortunately, some of these people have professional qualifications.

This type of misinformation can be dangerous to the public in two different ways:

1. The products or theories are inherently dangerous or injurious to health.
2. The products or theories are in themselves harmless, but people with serious health problems may fail to avail themselves for proper medical treatment, and opt to use the quack products or treatments instead.

While snake-oil and elixer salesmen have been around a long time, the modern era of health misinformation probably began with fascination over the vitamins. Moreover, erroneous attributes of vitamins have received so much publicity, that practically every household in the country has been affected. The public has been bombarded with misinformation to the point that misguided beliefs concerning vitamins can be considered part of a health folklore. Known as megavitamin or megadose therapy, it is commonly believed that excessive doses of vitamins will cure a number of common ailments, and/or give us more "pep" and energy. Vitamin A is often touted to be a cure for skin blemishes, the B vitamins are the "energy" vitamins, vitamin C is the anti-cold and flu vitamin, and vitamin E, of course, is the sexual fountain of youth.

These specific misconceptions probably have their roots in extrapolation of legitimate scientific information concerning what happens when these vitamins are deficient. In vitamin A deficiency, skin eruptions and dermatitis are one of several symptoms. Several of the B vitamins are essential components in the biochemistry of carbohydrate metabolism, and a deficiency therefore results in physical weakness and lack of energy. Vitamin C is involved in protein metabolism, and a deficiency of the vitamin results in the classic deficiency disease known as scurvy. Although the mechanisms are not clearly understood, it is known that people affected by scurvy are more susceptible to infectious diseases. Vitamin E is required for spermatogenesis, and a deficiency will result in reduced fertility and eventually testicular degeneration. In the female, a deficiency of vitamin E will result in the inability of the fertilized ovum to implant in the uterine wall.

Discovery of most of the vitamins and their functions has occurred relatively recently (within the last 50-60 years). Each discovery has been heralded by considerable publicity describing (in very general terms) the metabolic problems the compounds are able to correct. For example, when vitamin E was ultimately discovered, it was announced as the anti-sterility factor. Indeed, the scientific name of vitamin E is tocopherol, which is taken from the Greek words tocos, which means "birth", and phero, which means, "bring forth".

It is the nature of man to oversimplify, and so when vitamin E was announced as a cure for sterility, it wasn't long before the public began extrapolating on the powers of this new compound; "If in small doses it can cure sterility, then in massive doses it should probably cure impotency". While not intended as a double entendre, such thinking is purely a fantasy.

Vitamins are required in minute quantities for use in very complex biochemical reactions. Taking doses in excess of what is required for those functions simply is not beneficial. On the contrary, when vitamins (or most other nutrients, for that matter) are taken in substantial excess, they can be quite toxic. One of the most toxic is vitamin A. Extraordinarily heavy doses of vitamin A can cause bone deformation, nerve and brain damage, and death. For most vitamins, one must take man-made vitamin preparations in order to get enough for a toxicity to occur. Vitamin A is an exception, as livers of certain animal species contain very high level concentrations. Anthropologists have reported finding bone damage characteristic of vitamin A toxicity in the remains of human skeletons over one million years old (homo erectus/ Peking Man).[1] Likewise, Arctic explorers have been known to have suffered toxicities from eating Polar Bear liver. As one might expect, there have also been toxicities due to taking excessive levels of vitamin A via vitamin capsules.

Indeed, the taking of massive quantities of vitamins and minerals has become a major concern among health professionals. Concern has been increasing because in addition to the innocent misinformation spread through what has been termed the health folklore, the last few years have seen a rapid rise in purposefully fraudulent literature designed to promote sales of concentrated vitamin and mineral products.*

This type of literature has taken its toll. To cite some known instances of toxicities due to erroneous literature: A sixteen year old boy suffered serious brain damage after taking 50,000 I.U. of vitamin A over a 2½ year period, as a supposed cure for acne. As the result of a book on children's diets, an infant girl suffered nervous system damage and permanent growth retardation due to excessive vitamin A, and another infant girl was killed due to an overdose of potassium, as a supposed cure for colic. [2]

Fraudulent claims and scientific misinformation have been by no means restricted to vitamins and minerals. On the contrary, recognizing the public's concern for health, the health food charlatans have begun marketing a whole host of lucrative, but worthless products. The latest craze seems to be amino acid preparations.

Literature on these products describes them as being capable of curing everything from insomnia to arthritis. In some cases, these products contain vitamins, minerals, and herbs, in addition to amino acids.

One preparation which consists of a single amino acid, phenylalanine, has been said to be an appetite suppressant (for dieting), which functions on the brain. While phenylalanine is found in protein containing foods, it was said that it is better to take the pure form (the offered product), so it doesn't have to compete with other amino acids to get to the brain. The fact of the matter is that whenever a single or otherwise unbalanced group of amino acids are ingested, they are broken down and used for energy. That is, amino acids consist of a nitrogen containing (amine) group connected to a carbohydrate like carbon group. When amino acids are not needed for protein formation, the carbohydrate group is sent to the cells to be used as energy.

---

*In at least one case, the health food charlatans have even tried to create a new vitamin . . . vitamin B_{15}. A complete hoax, done for the purpose of selling a worthless product.

While the herbs contained in these types of preparations might be suspect, the amino acids (if chemically pure) are probably harmless.* Taking them will just add a few calories to the diet, and some extra nitrogen to the urine.

Reading the material on these products would almost be comical,** if it weren't for the fact that these con-men/hucksters often prey on the elderly and infirm. Degenerative diseases such as arthritis appear to be almost readymade for health food fraud. There are no legitimate cures, so the snake-oil salesmen have a very vulnerable market. This was driven home to me when I found that my father, terminally ill with Parkinson's Disease (a neurological disorder), had purchased a bottle of ribonucleic acid (RNA). Ribonucleic acid, of course, is a complex protein used in cellular reproduction, but is touted by current health food propaganda as a brain stimulent. In actuality, when ribonucleic acid is ingested, it is broken down into its amino acids like any other protein. Swallowing a capsule of purified RNA (if that is what the capsule actually contains) is like swallowing so much beefsteak. Indeed, all meats (and most vegetable foods) contain ribonucleic acid since they contain cells and cellular matter. The ribonucleic acid is broken down along with the rest of the proteins, and added to the body's amino acid pool.

In an almost emotional plea, Dr. Victor Herbert, the president of the American Society for Clinical Nutrition, has pointed out that the public must be brought to the realization that it is legal to lie about nutrition. The health food quacks are protected by the first ammendment. The only thing they cannot do, is put their claims on the label of the product they are selling. There are Food and Drug Laws against that. It is legal to make fraudulent claims about any sort of health food, vitamin, mineral, etc., as long as the claim does not appear on the bottle or package. Erroneous scientific data, ridiculous statements, and purposefully misleading claims are even legal to put on literature describing the product . . . as long as the literature appears on a shelf separate from the product.

If a health food salesperson makes some claims about a particular product, ask that they put it on the label. Ask them to write out whatever the product is supposed to do or cure, have them sign their name to it, and then tape it to the bottle. As Dr. Herbert has pointed out, they won't do it. If they do, they are

*If vitamins and minerals are present, one should beware of the levels.
**One amino acid product has been said to cure venereal disease.

in violation of federal Food and Drug Labeling Laws, and are subject to prosecution. Instead, they will probably try to give you a separate piece of literature.

Dr. Herbert has also pointed out that the public should be informed as to the existance of what are termed "diploma mill universities". These are institutions, sometimes registered with a state (but not accredited), that will grant mail-order BS, MS, and Ph.D. degrees in nutrition.[2] The text material used in these correspondence courses consists primarily of health food fad books and literature. These people, under the guise of having professional qualifications, then add to the health food literature with fad books and articles of their own.

However, in the author's opinion, it should also be pointed out, that some of the people authoring or selling these health fads, do indeed have legitimate professional training. At least one of the current popular diet books, labeled as "potentially dangerous", by the American Medical Association, was written by a physician. An earlier starvation type diet book which resulted in two known deaths, was also written by a physician. The amount of money in this thing is so big that even people sworn to professionalism have apparently had their morals corrupted.

As an animal nutritionist, for a long time I was hesitant about writing or publishing a book such as this one. My primary fears being that I would be criticized for my professional qualifications, and would be perceived to be someone else just trying to hop on the health fad bandwagon. However, as time went on it became clear that the health food quacks and diet gurus were continuing to gain ground. Legitimate, dedicated health professionals were speaking out, but not in a form that was accessible to the public. They were writing in the professional and scientific journals, or otherwise using text and vocabulary suited for readers with technical training. A few professionals were making the television talk shows, but by and large, the message was not getting to the public.

As an animal nutritionist I have come to understand the value and necessity of communication. For example, the manager of a 10,000 head feedlot has a very keen interest in nutrition. At $450/head, he has responsibility for a one time investment of 4.5 million dollars in cattle, and will spend about 4.6 million dollars a year on feed. He may not have formal training in the biological sciences, but he is unquestionably very interested in the technical aspects as they pertain to his feeding operation. In explaining the aspects of nutrition to him, they must not only be very detailed, but exceedingly clear. There is no room for error; just a 2% inefficiency or mistake will cost the man $92,000/year.

In the area of human nutrition, we don't have costs and figures like that to deal with . . . but we do have human life. However, it has been my observation that human health professionals rarely try to really communicate with their patients. They may say, "take two of these daily", or "eat more vegetables or complex carbohydrates", but there is usually no attempt to explain the technical details of their recommendations. They may say, "your blood triglycerides are too high, your blood pressure is too high, etc.", but rarely do they become involved in a detailed discussion. The physician or health professional typically doesn't feel the patient is capable of understanding the details.

It is my sincerest conviction that education is not synonymous with intelligence. Science is difficult to read or understand to a large extent because of specialized vocabulary . . . vocabulary that only those with training in the specific field would be readily conversant in. If, however, specialized vocabulary is replaced with everyday language, and if basic principles are explained in relation to things that can be readily identified with (rather than abstract), much of the public can be made to understand basic science.

With that in mind, I have attempted to write this book. While I realized that I would have some deficiency in specific areas of human nutrition, I felt I did have the necessary communicative skills. When you make your living explaining biological science to cowboys, you learn to communicate.

In preparation for this book, I spent over two years studying and reviewing literature on human nutrition. If I have an area of deficiency, it is in the intricacies of the biochemical pathways involved in digestion and intermediary metabolism. I am not a biochemist. Likewise, I would not be capable of discussing the biochemical fine points involved in animal nutrition. I do, however, consider myself very competent to design and implement practical nutrition and feeding programs for animals and livestock.

After an intensive period of study (coupled with an academic background), I now consider myself competent to explain the basic principles of human nutrition. In no way do I consider myself to be an "expert" in human nutrition. I do consider myself to be an exceedingly good communicator or teacher in the area of basic science. Communicative skills, plus a sound basic understanding of nutrition, is what I perceive to be the requirements for writing a book such as this. I sincerely believe that I have those require-ments, and that the writing of this book has been a public service. I recognize that there are a number of health professionals who will make light of my qualifications, but I do hope there will be others who recognize that someone must get the message accross.

SECTION I - DIET AND WEIGHT LOSS

Chapter 2   UNDERSTANDING HUNGER

(WHY WE BECOME AS HUNGRY OR HUNGRIER WHEN WE DO OFFICEWORK AS WHEN WE DO PHYSICAL WORK).

Hunger is what stands between many people and staying on a diet plan. It is often said that hunger is a test for willpower or self discipline. Actually, this is a rather crude or uneducated way of thinking or dealing with hunger. It is the author's opinion that if the dieter understands the physiological conditions that cause hunger, he or she can cope with it more easily.

As a simple explanation of hunger, one might say that hunger is Nature's way of telling us that we need to eat. This might be true if we were still living in a primitive environment, but it is not true in our modern society. In order to maintain maximum productivity, most of us must work with our brains, and let machines do the physical work.

The physiological mechanisms within the body that cause the hunger sensation, do not compensate for modern employment. Rather, our hunger mechanisms assume that in order to survive, we still must toil and forage all our waking hours. In essence, our physiological mechanisms are geared to the lifestyles of aboriginal peoples. Therefore our bodies tell us to eat whether we really need to or not.

Hunger mechanisms. There are two basic mechanisms that create the sensation of hunger. The first and most easily understood mechanism of sensation is caused by a series of stretch receptors in the stomach. As we eat and the stomach becomes distended, these receptors are stretched which creates a feeling of fullness.

The feeling of fullness, however, does not have the last word in telling our brain that we should or shouldn't continue eating. A far more important factor and indeed an overriding factor is the blood sugar level.

Blood sugar is the common name for glucose; a simple sugar which is the end product of most carbohydrate digestion. Glucose is the body's most readily usable form of energy, and the body closely monitors the blood glucose level at all times. This is very important since the brain and red blood cells can use only glucose for energy.

To hold us over between meals, glucose is stored in the liver and other tissues in a form known as glycogen. Glycogen is simply long chains of glucose held together by a weak chemical bond.

When the body deems it necessary that the blood glucose level be increased, hormones are secreted which in turn cause the release of glycogen.

The most well known of these hormones is adrenaline. As the reader is probably well aware, the secretion of adrenaline is primarily controlled by our emotions. If we are frightened or otherwise extremely excited, the body will deem it necessary to release large quantities of adrenaline, which in turn releases large quantities of glycogen/glucose. The increased level of glucose in the blood is largely responsible for the remarkable strength and abilities people often display when faced with life or death situations. Likewise, this is why the use of injected adrenaline* in athletic events, horseracing, etc. is strictly forbidden.

The other major hormone involved is known as glucogan. Physical exercise is the primary stimulus affecting the release of glucogan. The purpose, of course, is to replace the glucose burned up during exercise.

Obviously then, in order for the body to utilize stored glucose (glycogen), we must be physically or emotionally stimulated. In primeval societies, this is no problem. Most of the day the

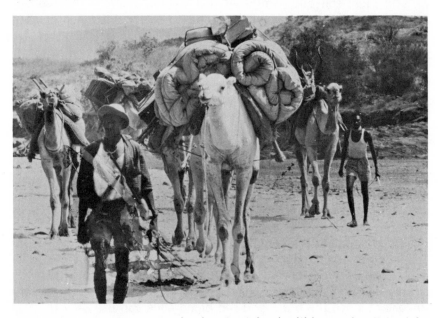

Figure 2-1. The hunger mechanism contained within us, is attuned for primeval existance. It assumes that we must toil all our waking hours, and does not compensate for modern employment.

*The medical term is epinepherine.

populace is engaged in hunting, fishing, or some other type of physical activity. But in our modern society, the majority of us are forced into sessile type endeavors. To society as a whole this yields a net benefit since we are more productive, but it leaves the individual stuck with employment that is usually not emotionally or physically stimulating. Because of this, for about 40 hours a week our bodies secrete very little adrenalin or glucogan, and therefore use very little of the glycogen/glucose reserves during that period.

Thus, about 10:00 AM and 3:00 PM, as our blood glucose levels begin to drop (glucose from the previous meal is used up), the body tells the brain that we need to eat, even though there is considerable reserve glucose readily available. We develop a substantial hunger, even though we have not exerted ourselves physically. Come mealtime, we are just as hungry as a day laborer who has burned up substantially more energy. His body tells him to eat because his glucose stores are used up and he needs to replace them; our bodies tell us to eat simply because our blood glucose levels are low. The laborer receives the stimulus to eat (hunger) because his blood glucose level is low, but it is low because there are no more stores to replace it. Our glucose is low because the body will not release the stores.

This puts us in a bad position. Our bodies are telling us to eat as much or nearly as much as the laborer. But if we actually eat that much, the energy that goes to replace the glucose stores in the laborer, will go to produce fat in us (since our glucose stores don't need replacing).

Skipping a meal. For three to four hours after hunger first strikes we will continue to experience hunger. After a while we will begin to feel weak. This is due to the lower glucose or energy level in the blood. Often a headache will develop, which is also due to a lack of glucose (lack of oxygen, as in asphyxia will also produce an intense headache).

If we do not eat, after a while the intense sensation of hunger will fade away. Likewise, we will gradually lose the feeling of weakness. This is because the metabolism of the body is shifting over to utilize stored fat. Proteins can be broken down to form glucose units, and so the body will begin breaking down body proteins for brain and red blood cell use. This is why starvation or malnutrition victims appear emaciated of the musculature as well as devoid of body fat. This is also why meal skipping or starvation dieting is a very poorly conceived method of weight control (Chapter 4).

Nutritional considerations. We need to remember that while we don't have the energy requirements of someone who labors all day long, we do have the same need for protein, vitamins, and minerals. What this means is that we need to eat foods that have a "high nutrient density". That is, foods that are rich in vitamins, minerals, and/or protein and fiber. We need to avoid foods that contain what are known as "empty calories". As explained in Chapter 6, these types of foods should be avoided not only for nutritional considerations, but also because they tend to intensify the hunger sensation as well.

Summary. The sensation of hunger is controlled by two primary mechanisms. Stretch receptors in the stomach tell us when the stomach is empty or full. A much more powerful mechanism, is the blood sugar or glucose level. The brain and the red blood cells require glucose for normal functioning. The body therefore closely monitors the blood glucose level. When the blood glucose level falls, the brain sends out a signal in the form of the hunger sensation. If we do not eat (skip a meal), proteins within the body are broken down to form glucose (to supply the brain and red blood cells).

Hormones secreted within the body can cause stored glucose to be released. However, these hormones require that we be physically or emotionally stimulated before they can be released. For those of us with sedentary occupations, these stimulae typically do not occur during working hours. Therefore at meal time, we typically have as great an appetite as someone who has been physically active. A laborer will have an appetite because his glucose reserves have been depleted; we will have an appetite because our reserves have not been released. While we don't have the same energy requirement as the laborer, we have essentially the same requirement for protein, vitamins, and minerals. We must therefore avoid foods that contain "empty calories" (sugar, cornstarch, and flour). These foods should be avoided not only for nutritional reasons, but also because they tend to intensify the sensation of hunger (between meals) (Chapter 6).

Chapter 3 WHY CALORIE COUNTING CAN BE MISLEADING

Calorie charts and subsequent counting has been the mainstay of most diet plans. The problem with calorie counting is that the caloric values given for different foods are primarily based on laboratory or calculated values. These values do not take rate of digestion into consideration, which can actually be more important than the caloric value. Foods that are digested very quickly (such as sugar) can actually be more fattening than foods that may be higher in calories, but are digested more slowly. This is essentially because slowly digested foods give the body time to burn off the calories they release, whereas quickly digested foods do not. Quickly digested foods release all their calories in a short time span, and what is not needed for energy, is transformed into fat.

The term calorie means the amount of energy required to heat one gram of water one degree Centigrade. To measure the caloric content of foods a device known as a bomb calorimeter is usually used. This is a piece of equipment which burns a measured amount of a foodstuff in an atmosphere of pure oxygen (to ensure complete burning). The heat given off is measured and thus the number of calories in the food is determined. Fats are said to contain 2.25 times as many calories as carbohydrates since they release that much more energy when burned in a calorimeter.

Obviously, the human digestive tract does not utilize an electric spark in an atmosphere of pure oxygen to break down foods. The body uses a number of digestive enzymes and processes to "burn" (oxydize) energy foods. Besides the obvious mechanical difference (between a calorimeter and the digestive tract) the main difference of importance to dieting, is the length of time required for digestion. A calorimeter can burn the energy from all human foods in a matter of seconds . . . in a human digestive tract the time required for digestion can vary from a few minutes up to 12 hours.

Refined carbohydrates such as table sugar and bleached flour are digested very quickly. Indeed, digestion of refined starches (white flour) begins the minute they are placed in the mouth. Saliva contains an enzyme which begins breaking them down even before they reach the stomach. When refined carbohydrates do reach the stomach, they don't stay there very long. Unless the stomach also contains a large amount of fat or protein, refined carbohydrates are passed to the small intestine in a matter of minutes. Final digestion and absorption takes place in the upper end of the small intestine that connects to the stomach (duodenum). For highly refined carbohydrates, absorption usually occurs very quickly.

Of all the carbohydrates in the human diet, common table sugar is the most quickly digested (and therefore the most fattening). We are all familiar with the quick "pick-me-up" we experience from drinking sugar laden soda pop or eating candy. If you have ever seen a diabetic going through a temporary shortage of blood sugar (hypoglycemia), you know just how quickly sugar can be digested. A diabetic can be trembling and shaking . . . drink a glass of sugar water, and stop trembling within 3 to 5 minutes!

It is because sugar and other refined carbohydrates are digested so quickly, that they can be particularly "fattening". Carbohydrates are all broken down to form glucose, a simple sugar that is used as a primary energy source in the body. The body is very sensitive to the glucose level in the blood. When the level becomes elevated (after eating a candy bar, etc.), insulin is secreted which pulls the excess glucose out of the blood. Some of the glucose is stored as a carbohydrate reserve (known as glycogen), and the rest is synthesized into body fat.

Unrefined carbohydrates such as potatoes or whole cereal grains, however, are not broken down and digested nearly as quickly. They aren't broken down as quickly because they have not been refined, or otherwise artificially processed. That is, the starch contained in unprocessed carbohydrate food is typically surrounded by what is known as a protein matrix. The starch is contained in a granule, which is surrounded by a relatively tough protein coating (Figures 3-1 & 3-2). Because the protein coating complexes the starch, making digestion more difficult, unrefined carbohydrates are often referred to as "complex carbohydrates".

During the processing of sugar, flour, or cornstarch, the protein coating is removed. As mentioned, this protein coating is actually a barrier to digestion. With the coating removed, the digestive enzymes within the body are able to break down and digest the carbohydrate much more quickly. As a result, their energy is released more quickly and they are therefore much more likely to cause the synthesis of body fat.

Dietary fats take even longer to digest. Fat molecules are difficult to break down and therefore stay in the stomach much

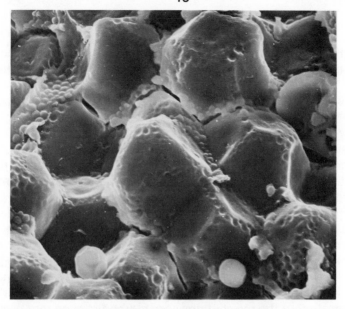

Figure 3-1. Starch contained in cereal grains. Note the heavy structuring of the protein coating that surrounds the starch granules. This coating forms a barrier to digestion, thereby slowing down the release of the energy (from the starch). When the starch has been removed and refined (as in Figure 3-2, below) it no longer has its protective coating. Therefore the digestive enzymes are able to break it down much more quickly . . . thereby releasing its energy much more quickly, and making it much more likely to be used for synthesis of body fat.
(Figure 3-1, corn magnified 1750X, courtesy Dr. Carl Hoseney, Kansas State University.
Figure 3-2, isolated corn starch, magnified 2000X, courtesy Dr. Don Wagner, Oklahoma State University.)

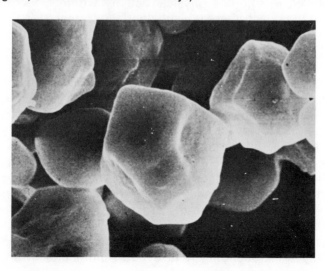

longer than carbohydrates (that is why greasy foods tend to cause indigestion and discomfort). When released from the stomach, fats are mixed with enzymes secreted from the gall bladder and pancreas for further degradation. Final absorption takes place at the far end of the small intestine (Figure 19-1, p. 170). This process normally takes several hours to complete.

What this means to dieting, is that unless we are dealing with an immobile hospital patient, etc., there is more opportunity or time to burn off the energy released from dietary fats or complex carbohydrates than refined carbohydrates such as sugar. This means that the caloric values put on foods can be misleading in terms of dieting. For example, the caloric values for a hamburger are approximately the same as for a slice of meringue pie. However, the hamburger isn't nearly as "fattening" as the pie. The energy or calories in the hamburger are coming primarily from the fat in the meat and the flour in the bun. Flour, of course, is a refined carbohydrate, but the pie contains corn starch (an even more refined carbohydrate), and is loaded with sugar (the most quickly digested food in the human diet).

Either out of an innate desire for the sweet taste, or possibly as a conditioning created by the fact that nearly all prepared foods are laced with sugar, most people have a hard time resisting sweets. Thus, when following a typical "calorie counter" diet, and given the choice of a staple food or a sweet, many people will pass up milk, potatoes, and / or butter at mealtime, but will eat the dessert . . . thinking that as long as they stay within a predetermined caloric intake level, there is no difference. Unless they are going to be involved in rigorous physical activity within a few minutes after eating the sweet, there is a substantial difference.

The question, "What is the value of fats vs. refined carbo-hydrates", cannot be answered in simple mathematic terms. Like all disciplines in the study of biology, nutrition and dieting is an inexact science. To arrive at a value will call for judgement as well as mathematics.

If we have someone who is continuously engaged in strenuous activity, the 2.25 factor for fats vs. carbohydrates is probably appli-cable. Likewise, all carbohydrates could be considered equal. If we are involved in sedentary occupations, however, fatty foods (butter, hamburger, fried potatoes, etc.) will not carry as great a fattening potential as the 2.25 energy factor would indicate. Likewise, complex carbohydrates are going to be much less fat-tening than refined carbohydrates. In the very normal situation most of us are faced with . . . where we can partake in physical activity only after spending 4 to 8 hours immobile in an office, refined carbohydrates have much more "fattening potential" than complex carbohydrates, or foods high in fat.

Notice that the terms <u>energy factor</u> and <u>fattening potential</u> are kept separate. Fattening potential in a food can change depending upon the physical activity after the food is eaten, but the energy factor never changes. A food always contains a given number of calories. It is how quickly those calories are given off, and the lifestyle of the individual that determines the "fattening potential". For example, in the preceding paragraph it was stated that for a person with a normal 9 to 5 office job, refined carbohydrates (sugar and flour) have a greater "fattening potential" than complex carbohydrates or foods high in fats. Explained in more detail, this essentially means that a person who eats a fried egg, a couple slices of bacon or sausage, and a slice of buttered whole wheat toast for breakfast, will stand less chance of getting fat than a person who eats a couple of sweet rolls and a cup of coffee. Likewise, the person who eats a hamburger steak, french fries, green salad, and a glass of milk for lunch, will stand less chance of getting fat than the person who eats a couple of sandwiches (on white bread) and a soda pop. As explained earlier, this is because refined carbohydrates will be totally digested and released during the time we spend in the office. Therefore, what energy is not burned up will be stored in the body (primarily as fat). Unrefined carbohydrates and fat take more time to digest and release their energy over a longer time span, thereby giving us the opportunity to burn off some of the energy during an afterwork tennis game, jogging program, etc. In addition, people who eat foods that release their energy more slowly will have a more constant blood sugar level, and therefore will not become as hungry between meals (Chap. 6). That is, they will be less prone to eat between meals.

Summary. The caloric content of foods is determined by laboratory analysis. The device used is known as a bomb calorimeter, which utilizes an electric spark in an atmosphere of pure oxygen. This device can "digest" all foods in a matter of seconds.

Digestion in the human digestive tract takes much longer and is quite variable. Highly refined carbohydrates such a sugar can be digested as quickly as 15 minutes, whereas fats may take up to 8 hours. Because refined carbohydrates tend to release their energy more quickly, there is a greater chance the body will absorb the energy for the formation of fat. Foods that are digested more slowly, tend to release their energy at a slower rate, which gives the body more time to "burn it off". Therefore while some foods may have similar caloric values, they may be quite different in terms of their "fattening potential".

Chapter 4 DIETING TO MAKE US MORE ATTRACTIVE, RATHER THAN JUST THIN

As a nation, current public opinion would indicate a seeming obscession with sex. Ignoring promiscuity, and the commercial exploitation of sex, psychologists do tell us that for a marriage to remain truly viable, there must be an active sex life. Obviously, in order for this to occur both partners must be attracted to each other. Those of us brought up in more conservative environments may not like to think about or discuss sex quite so graphically, but in reality we know the psychologists are probably correct. In countries where attitudes are outwardly more Puritan, the situation is usually that if Papa has a big fat Mama at home . . . he usually has a mistress or two somewhere else.

Likewise, while we may not want to say it openly (or even admit it to ourselves), we would all like to be "sexy". When we say we want to lose weight, what we are really saying is that we want to be more attractive. At this point (right from the beginning), many dieters get their intentions confused. They think of weight loss as being synonymous with becoming more attractive. If the reader gets only one thing out of this chapter, it should be that weight loss and becoming more attractive are not necessarily synonymous. Weight loss is usually a part of becoming more attractive . . . but slender is not necessarily sexy. (Don Knotts and Phyllis Diller are quite slender, but they would hardly be considered sexy.)

Sexual attractiveness implies a robust, vivacious glow of health. Starvation dieting, diet pills, gimmics and fads will not impart a robust glow of health. Only proper diet, exercise, and rest will do that. The following is a discussion drawn from subjects discussed in more detail in other chapters . . . tying all the subjects together to help us achieve the goal we are really seeking.

From the previous discussion the first thing that should be evident is that dieting alone is not sufficient. Anyone truly concerned about his or her health, well being, or physical appearance, must also partake in an exercise program. Indeed, one must coordinate his or her diet program to fit their exercise regimen. Choosing the proper diet is discussed at length in Chapter 6 and the proper exercise program in Chapter 8. The point the author wishes to make in this chapter is that there must be both.

Open up any magazine with a broad readership and you will

find numerous advertisements for gimmics, gadgets, pills, and books that all promise the same thing. They all promise something for nothing; lose weight without dieting; flatten your tummy without exercise; eat less without feeling hungry; become powerfully muscled in just 20 minutes a day; etc., etc.

American ingenuity has made this country what it is. However, there are no short cuts to health. Medical science has produced drugs and techniques to correct individual ailments or diseases, but there is no single pill, gadget, fufu powder, or even diet that will bring overall health. To reiterate, the only way we can truly enhance our physical appearance is through the adoption of a lifestyle that permits a reasonable amount of exercise, proper diet, and rest.

Starvation dieting is probably the most serious mistake made by people who want to be more attractive. Starvation dieting detracts from our appearance in two ways: 1. it reduces muscle tissue as well as fat tissue; and 2. it leaves us too weak to exercise or perform our usual physical chores with the same vigor . . . thereby reducing muscle tone further.

Women may underestimate the value of muscle size and tone, but ladies, please remember that it is the musculature that puts shape in the legs, hips, and torso. What separates Juliet Prowse from Phyllis Diller is not a matter of pounds, but a matter of musculature (which to a large extent is most certainly due to a substantial difference in exercise regimens).

As described in Chap. 2, starvation dieting forces the body to breakdown body proteins (muscles). This is primarily because the brain and red blood cells cannot utilize fat for energy, they must have glucose (blood sugar). Glucose cannot be synthesized from fat but it can be synthesized from amino acids. Also, a certain amount of protein is needed to repair and maintain vital organs. The body will therefore pull protein away from non-vital areas (legs, hips, arms, chest, etc.), for use in the heart, brain, and digestive and respiratory tracts.

A modification of the starvation diet has been the so called high protein diet. Whenever a weight reduction plan is begun, it is always good advice to increase the level of protein. But to eat nothing but protein is both ill advised and dangerous. The idea that eating nothing but protein will force the body to utilize only fat stores for energy is catagorically wrong. Instead, the body will attempt to meet its energy needs from dietary protein by breaking it down to form glucose. As by-products of that process, nitrogenous products are formed which can place a stress on the liver and kidneys. Although usually complicated by other deficiency problems, if carried to extremes, the situation can be fatal. At any rate, it doesn't create a radiant glow of health.

Probably the most common type of starvation dieting is meal skipping. This type of diet plan (if it can be called that), usually yields very poor results for a variety of reasons. Again, the body protein breakdown to provide glucose during the fasting period is a problem. For a given amount of food, several small meals are preferable to fewer larger meals. Fewer larger meals release their energy over a shorter time period which limits the time the body has to burn the energy up. Therefore there will be more energy available for fat deposition. This is particularly true if the meal that is skipped is breakfast or lunch. In addition, if breakfast or lunch is skipped, the person will not feel as strong or energetic during the daylight hours, and will therefore not burn up as much energy as they otherwise would. After dinner is eaten in the evening, there is usually little opportunity to burn off energy.

Summary. Losing weight and becoming more attractive are not always synonymous. Radical forms of dieting or weight loss will debilitate the musculature, as well as reduce body fat.

The brain and red blood cells cannot use fat as a source of energy. Proteins can be broken down to form glucose, which is the form of energy required by the brain and red blood cells. Starvation type dieting (including meal skipping) thereby forces the body to breakdown muscle tissue. The end result is an overall body debilitation, rather than just reduction of excess fat. Starvation dieting also greatly reduces desire to participate in exercise programs, further reducing muscle shape and tone.

Physical attractiveness is very much dependent upon the shapliness of the musculature. This is just as true for women as it is men. Crash diets will not result in the most desireable musculature. Moreover, the term sex appeal can best be described as a radiant glow of health and vitality. Crash dieting will not convey a radiant glow of health . . . only proper nutrition, exercise, and rest will do that.

Chapter 5 THE REVOLUTIONARY UNBALANCED DIET

In our modern society the quickest way to get attention (especially media coverage) is to do something contrary to accepted standards. Moreover, in the area of technology, we have become conditioned to rapid advancement and revolutionary change.

In assessing the value of new ideas, we must recognize that we cannot computer program our bodies to accept a new fuel or utilize an electronic ignition system. Our bodies are designed to function in a certain manner, and if we attempt to tamper with the way it functions . . . we are courting trouble.

Such is the case with the fad diets. In reality, the "revolutionary" diets are nothing more than unbalanced diets, that someone is always trying to promote as "a new scientific breakthrough". As far as science is concerned, Grandmother knew a lot more about nutrition when she told us to eat everything on our plate, than the modern day diet gurus that tell us not to eat carbohydrate, or eat only protein, or only fish, or vegetables, etc., etc.

The thing we must remember is that most of the fad diets will work. Anytime we restrict our intake of calorie containing foods, whether they be carbohydrate, fat, or protein . . . we will lose weight. The thing that we must also keep in mind is that dietary extremes are basically unhealthy.

As any good home economist or dietitian will tell us, it is important to eat a wide variety of foods. There are a myriad of reasons for this, but one of the most basic is that many foods contain potentially toxic compounds. For example, vegetables contain relatively high levels of nitrates. Nitrates, of course, can be toxic at high concentrations. Also, nitrates can combine with certain protein-like compounds (amines) to form nitrosamines, which are well known to cause stomach cancer (see p. 114). In Japan, where there is heavy reliance on vegetables and fish (very high in free amines), there is also a high stomach cancer rate.

Does this mean we should be afraid of vegetables? Absolutely not. Indeed, vegetables are a vital ingredient in a well balanced diet. Vegetables are a good source of fiber, which is believed to be protective of dysfunctions of the large bowel. In the U.S., where there is a general lack of fiber in the diet, there is also a relatively high rate of cancer of the colon (p. 116), and diverticulitis.

But should we be afraid of consuming vegetables with protein, especially fish? No, not as long as we eat potato, tomato, or some type of fruit at the same time. Vitamin C prevents nitrates from combining with amines, and therefore if we eat a balanced diet we have nothing to be concerned about. A diet of meat, potato, and vegetables will give us our protein, fiber to protect us from bowel problems, and vitamin C to protect us from cancer of the stomach.

But can't we get along without carbohydrate? This is a very basic question since most diets recommend reducing or eliminating carbohydrate. The answer depends on what kind of carbohydrate we are talking about. If we are talking about highly refined carbohydrates such as table sugar, the answer is an unqualified yes. Indeed, in the diet chapter (Chap. 6) of this book, reducing or eliminating sugar is the first recommendation. The human race got along fine without sugar for centuries . . . it has only been the last 200 years that refined sugar has been part of the diet.

If we are talking about what are known as complex carbohydrates (potatoes, brown rice, whole cereal grains, fruit, etc.), the answer is probably not. Energy must come from somewhere. If it doesn't come from carbohydrate, then it must come from protein or fat.

Many diets recommend a relatively high protein regimen, and many dieters believe that protein is less fattening than carbo-

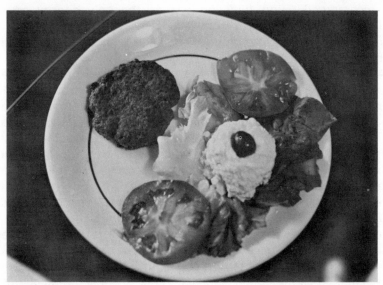

Figure 5-1. Many dieters believe that protein is less fattening than carbohydrate. That is not true. Protein and carbohydrate have the same energy value, and substituting protein for carbohydrate doesn't reduce caloric intake, but does place an extra burden on the kidneys.

hydrate. The thinking being that protein is used for muscle growth and maintenance, whereas carbohydrate is for energy or fat production. The fact of the matter is that protein is used for muscle growth and maintenance only up to what is actually needed for that purpose. After that requirement is met, the excess will be broken down for energy, and/or fat production. By laboratory values protein actually contains more calories than carbohydrate (about 5.5 Calories/gram for protein vs. about 4 Calories/gram for carbohydrate). However, there is some energy expended in breaking down protein, which results in protein having about the same net value as carbohydrate.

To eat a high protein diet means the liver and kidneys are going to have to process a lot more nitrogen than usual. Whether this is detrimental isn't known with any real certainty. There were some deaths on the so called liquid protein diet, but the people were essentially on a starvation diet, so other factors were probably involved. At any rate, it would not seem prudent to overburdon our kidneys with excess nitrogen.

If we don't get our energy from carbohydrate, or protein, then (of course) it must come from fat. Indeed, there are fad diets that recommend using fats and oils as the only energy source (excluding all carbohydrate from the diet). The theory is that by forcing the body to utilize only fat for energy, it will mobilize and use body fat at a faster rate.

Although the theory has never actually been proven, scientifically it is an interesting idea. The problem, is that it creates a potentially dangerous physiological condition. Normally, there is a small amount of carbohydrate used in the biochemical process used to burn fat for energy. When carbohydrate is not available, fat is transformed into acetone and two similar compounds, collectively known as ketone bodies. The ketones are then burned via a different biochemical process that does not require carbohydrate. Apparently because the use of ketones is not normally used as a major source of energy, the ability to utilize them is somewhat limited. If reliance upon ketones is prolonged, excess ketones can begin to accumulate in the blood, creating a condition known as ketosis. This changes the acidity of the blood, creating what is known as metabolic acidosis. This is the same mechanism involved in diabetic coma. In the case of the diabetic, carbohydrate is present, but there is no insulin to pull it out of the blood for use in the cells . . . so the body is forced to use ketone bodies for fuel. Likewise, this is one of the primary mechanisms involved in death by starvation.

Vitamins and minerals. In addition to supplying carbohydrate, protein, and fiber, a balanced diet is, of course, also necessary to ensure that we get the vitamins and minerals that are required. As the reader is probably well aware, some of the food groups contain vitamins and minerals that cannot be obtained in adequate amounts unless that specific food group is included in the diet. Examples would be vitamin B_{12} from meat, calcium from dairy products, vitamin K from green vegetables, etc.

What the reader may not be aware of is that some food groups are required for efficient digestion of vitamins and minerals actually contained in other food groups. The best example of this is iron. Iron in contained in many vegetables, and is often included as a supplementary ingredient in bread. However, unless a meat product is included in the diet, the digestibility of iron from vegetable sources is very poor. If meat is not included, iron availability is only about 20-40% what it would otherwise be. This is very important since iron is usually marginal in most peoples' diets anyway. (Pregnant women usually cannot meet their iron requirement without supplementation.)

Summary. There is no substitute for a well balanced diet. The fad diets that claim to be "scientific breakthroughs", are not that at all. This does not mean that many of them will not work. Anytime energy containing foods are restricted (be they carbohydrate, fat, or protein), weight loss will occur. It is important to realize, however, that nutritional imbalances can be dangerous, and are usually unhealthy. The intelligent person should realize that a well balanced diet, with a reasonable restriction of energy containing foods (such as refined carbohydrates), in the long run is a much healthier, more effective approach. (The next chapter will explain such a plan).

Chapter 6   AN EFFECTIVE DIET PLAN

To be truly effective, a diet plan should do more than just take weight off. A good diet plan should be designed to keep weight off after the initial dieting period, and as explained in chapter 4, it should make us look more attractive, not just thin.

The initial loss of weight is the easiest part of any diet plan. A pound of fat is the equivalent of about 3,500 Calories, so all we need do is reduce our intake about 500 Calories per day, and we will lose about 1 lb. per week. If we are ambitious, a reduction of 1,000 Calories per day will result in a loss of 2 lbs. per week. (Two pounds per week is considered as the maximum reduction that should be attempted without the close supervision of a physician.[3])

As explained in the previous chapter, some of the fad diets will result in weight reduction. - However, as was also pointed out, most of these diets are potentially dangerous as they create serious dietary imbalances. In addition to the immediate health hazards, this type of thinking is bad as it makes it difficult to keep from regaining weight after the initial "crash" period. That is, by placing emphasis on radical ideas or restrictions instead of sound nutritional practices, most people are naturally prone to go back to the lifestyle and eating patterns that made them overweight in the first place.

There are also a lot of diet pills and other gimmicks. Some if them work, and some of them don't. Those that work either speed up the metabolism (burn up more energy), or suppress the appetite. Any drug that monkeys around with the body's metabolism or nervous system (hunger response) is potentially dangerous. Aside from the danger (and habit forming potential) of these drugs, they are bad in that they become a crutch. They teach the dieter to rely on something artificial, rather than good basic nutrition. Therefore, as with the fad diets, when he or she goes off the drug, they return to their old dietary habits.

The ideal diet plan is one that teaches sound basic nutrition while allowing the individual to gradually adjust his or her dietary patterns and lifestyle to afford weight loss. In this way, after the desired weight loss is achieved, there is no problem in keeping the weight off.

This is the type of concept that will be presented in this chapter. Rather than make any radical changes in the beginning, it is the author's opinion that a more gradual approach is more likely to be successful in the long run. That is, will enable the dieter to keep the weight off permanently.

BASIC PREMISE. The basic premise behind the diet plan that will be presented here, is that most people do not need to restrict their intake of basic foodstuffs in order to lose or maintain a desired weight. Except in cases of obvious overeating, the restriction or substitution of condiments and drinks which consist of what are typically called "empty calories", along with a moderate increase in physical activity, will afford the necessary weight control.

In terms of the four basic food groups (meat and poultry; fruit and vegetables; grains and starches; and dairy products), most people do not overeat. What causes them to gain weight is the amount of unnecessary high calorie snack or dessert type foods and drinks they consume. These types of foods are not only high in calories, but more importantly, are very high in what are known as refined carbohydrates (white flour, cornstarch, and sugar).

As discussed in chap. 3, for a given caloric value, refined carbohydrates (sugar in particular) can be more "fattening" than other foods such as complex carbohydrates (potatoes, whole cereal grains, etc.), proteins, and fats. They can be more "fattening" if physical exertion of some kind does not take place shortly after ingestion. That is, the energy contained in sugar is released within 5 to about 30 minutes, and unless there is some activity to burn that energy up, most of it will probably be converted to fat. In contrast, dietary fats, take 4 to about 8 hours to digest, so the energy is released much more slowly, and therefore there is more opportunity to burn the energy up. (Complex carbohydrates would be intermediate, depending upon the type, degree of cooking, and the amount eaten.)

FIRST STEP

The first phase of this diet plan is to begin cutting down on "empty calorie" foods. For the most part this means reducing or eliminating foods with a high sugar content. This is the most important part of the diet plan. It is not only the first step toward weight reduction, but it is also the crucial element in the ability to keep from regaining weight.

In achieving this phase of the program, don't try and do it all at once. It is not a test of your willpower. Rather, it must become a part of your lifestyle. All of us have an innate craving for sweets, and making an abrupt change will not reduce our desire for sugar. Rather, all it will do is create an intense craving. At some point in time, we are likely to "break" and go back to our old ways.

It is far better to set realistic goals and achieve them without undue self-deprivation. For example, if we are used to eating a doughnut or candy bar during morning and afternoon coffee breaks, make your first goal to substitute less fattening foods. Continue drinking soda pop, or eating desserts during meals, but eliminate candy and sugary foods during mid-morning and afternoon snacks. If you like, substitute a piece of fruit.

Sweets to substitute . Fruit, of course, contains sugar, but it is primarily in the form of fructose. Fructose does not trigger an insulin response, and takes much longer to metabolise than sucrose (table sugar). Insulin is involved in the initiation of fat synthesis, and this coupled with the rapid assimilation of glucose makes sucrose much more fattening. In addition, the total amount of sugar is much lower than commercially prepared candies and confections.

Aside from the difference in sugars and sugar content, the starch contained in fruit is much less fattening than the starch contained in most candies and pastries. The starch contained in commercially prepared sweets is usually in the form of flour or corn starch, which are what are known as highly refined carbohydrates. That is, they have had almost all the fiber removed. This makes them capable of being rapidly digested and metabolized. Again, anything that can be rapidly digested is prone to be fattening when we are not physically active (to burn off the energy).

The starch contained in fruit is in the form of complex carbohydrates. Since it has not been finely ground, the starch is much less available for rapid digestion. That is, starch in foods is normally present in granules, which are usually surrounded by a protein or fiber matrix. This matrix constitutes a barrier to digestion, and thereby increases the length of time it takes to digest the starch contained in it. Whenever starch has been finely ground, as in flour and corn starch, the protective matrix is physically broken, and thus the starch is readily exposed to digestive enzymes, and is subsequently capable of being digested very rapidly (see Figure 3-1 & 2).

Further reductions in sweets. Once you have adjusted to not eating candy or other sweets, take another step toward eliminating "empty calories". If you're used to drinking soda pop several times a day, cut down on the amount. For example, if you normally consume two bottles or cans of soda pop a day, reduce your consumption to one can or bottle. Try substituting fruit juice instead. After you get used to a nutritious drink such as orange juice, grape juice, etc., it won't be long before you'll want to substitute it for soda pop all the time.

Some people will want to substitute diet soft drinks. It can be argued that these products contain essentially no calories, whereas fruit juices do contain some food energy. In my opinion, it is better to shun all types of soda pop since the sweetness in diet drinks is designed to be equal to regular soda pop. The idea here is to cut down on sweets as well as calories.

By experience I can tell you that once you break the habit of consuming sweets, the desire for them lessens. After you get in the habit of eating nothing sweeter than fruit, the thought of eating candy or drinking soda pop actually becomes mildly nauseating.

Desserts. After eliminating candy, soda pop, and related items between meals, the next step is to cut down on desserts and other sugary foods eaten during meals. This is not as easy as cutting down on candy and soda pop. Cherry pie, apple cobbler, ice cream, nutbreads, etc. contain nutritious foods as well as sugar, and are therefore psychologically more difficult to turn down than simple junk food.

To cope with this problem, my advice is to consume these types of foods only when prepared at home. As explained in chapter 17, most desserts and related items can be made with a fraction of the sugar used in most commercial recipes. In most cases, using half to one-third the sugar actually makes the items more tasty. The full flavor of the ingredients comes through, without being drowned out by excess sugar.

In addition to reduced sugar, most of these items can be made with whole wheat or stone ground flour instead of white flour. Whole wheat flour contains the fiber (bran) which is removed from white flour, and stone ground flour not only contains the fiber, but is a much coarser product. Coarseness and fiber both tend to slow down the rate at which digestion occurs, and therefore gives us more opportunity to burn the calories off, before they are synthesized into fat.

Once you get used to eating these type homemade and more

flavorful desserts, similar foods prepared with high levels of sugar will taste sickening sweet.

PROBLEMS ASSOCIATED WITH CUTTING DOWN ON SWEETS

Cutting down on sweets is not easy. There is more to it than just the sweet taste. Sugar actually changes our metabolism. As explained graphically on p. 80, sugar actually increases the metabolic rate and respiratory quotient.

In addition, it is my belief that a constant intake of sugar impairs the ability of the body to mobilize stored carbohydrate (glycogen). What this means is that when someone reduces their intake of sugar, they will become much hungrier between meals. More importantly, a physiological feeling of weakness will come over the individual . . . a "sinking" type of feeling.

As explained in Chapter 2, low blood glucose is one of the primary determinants of the onset of hunger. Glucose is one of the componets of sugar. Sugar is digested very rapidly, and there-fore it has the ability to rapidly elevate the blood glucose level. This is why we typically lose our appetite shortly after eating a candy bar, or other sugary food.

Conversely, when it has been a while since we have eaten a glucose containing food, we get hungry. There is a physiological mechanism within the body that is supposed to moderate this situation. When the blood glucose level becomes low, a hormone known as glucogon is secreted from the pancreas. The function of this hormone is to cause the body's stored form of glucose (known as glycogen), to be broken down and released into the bloodstream.

It is my belief that when the body gets used to a constant influx of sugar, the hormonal release mechanism for glycogen becomes less sensitive to blood glucose levels. When the blood glucose level drops to a low level, the body simply "waits" for its usual mid-morning or mid-afternoon charge of sugar (rather than attempting to release stored glucose). This intensifies the sensation of hunger, and the feeling of muscular weakness.

I must point out that this theory has never been proven scientif-ically. To the best of my knowledge, it has never even been exam-ined. I have arrived at it soley through personal observation.

Like most Americans, I used to consume a large amount of sugar. When I started cutting down (abruptly), I found myself becoming excruciatingly hungry. Hunger that included a feeling of weakness almost to the point of trembling. As time went on, the intensity of hunger between meals began to decline. Ultimately the sensation of hunger became reduced to a modest level, and the feeling of extreme muscular weakness no longer occurs to anywhere near the same degree. It is my sincerest belief that the reason is that the body can learn to moderate blood glucose levels - which it doesn't have to do (to the same extent) on a high sugar diet. When the body gets a slug of sugar water or a bolus of sugary goo every two or three hours, there really isn't as great a need to mobilize stored glycogen.

I believe this theory to be true because of the documented ability of the body to adapt to differing dietary conditions. For example, it is well known that when certain required nutrients such as vitamins and minerals are taken in excess, the body becomes much less efficient at digesting and recycling them.

Related directly to glucose metabolism is the well known phenomenon of "carbohydrate loading", practiced by athletes. As those involved in athletics are aware, it is a common practice for athletic teams and individuals to use this principle to extend their endurance. Several days prior to a game or althletic meet, the participant eats no carbohydrate, only protein and fats. This "starves" the body for glucose. Just before the athletic event, a large meal comprised soley of carbohydrate is eaten. Suddenly supplied with carbohydrate, the body reacts by storing an extraordinarily large amount of it as glycogen (storage form of glucose). Obviously this gives the athlete a greater amount of energy to draw on, which results in greater endurance. It has been estimated that the amount of glycogen can actually be doubled by this practice.[4]*

It therefore seems reasonable to conclude that if the body can respond to an absence of glucose, it can likewise respond to a surplus. That is, instead of storing an increased amount, it can store (and release) a reduced amount. I believe this to be true because whenever I break my diet and begin eating ice cream, drinking soda pop, etc., the same thing reoccurs . . . intense hunger sensations, feeling of weakness, headaches, etc.

Gradual withdrawal from sugar. Because sugar apparently changes the body's regulation of glucose, it is much better to gradually eliminate it from the diet. There is no evidence that an abrupt elimination would cause a normal person any visible harm, but it is usually best not to stress the body to any great extent.

---

*The long term effects of this practice are not known, but presumably it is not a healthy practice. Potential problems include stress on the kidney and liver, as well as possible abnormal cholesterol metabolism.

A gradual reduction of sugar would save the individual the intense hunger that would typify an abrupt elimination, and therefore make it easier to stay on the diet. An abrupt elimination would create an intense craving for sweets, whereas a gradual reduction would actually reduce the craving.

SECOND STEP

After vowing to reduce the amount of sugar in the diet, the next step is to begin to increase physical activity. The purpose in exercising is not only to burn up calories, but to moderate or reduce the hunger level.

This second purpose is often misunderstood. Most people are of the opinion that exercise increases hunger. This is true only for prolonged muscular activity, such as several hours of weightlifting. Light or moderate exercise actually tends to reduce hunger.

As explained in the previous section (and Chap. 2), blood glucose levels are a major factor in regulating hunger. When blood glucose levels decline, the sensation of hunger occurs. Exercise tends to cause the release of hormones which in turn causes the release of glycogen (the storage form of glucose) into the blood.

Therefore, by moderating the blood glucose level, exercise tends to moderate the sensation of hunger as well. Knowing this, we can utilize exercise to make cutting down on sugar easier. When we feel the need for a snack, walk around the block, do a set of pushups, etc., instead. This really will take the edge off of our appetite (as well as burn off calories).

If we are used to eating sugary snacks, it is important to remember that exercise will not be able to totally eliminate the hunger sensation. But it will take the edge off of it. If we practice a gradual reduction of sugar (rather than an abrupt elimination), light exercise should make the hunger sensations at least tolerable.

Heavy, prolonged exercise, of course, will tend to increase the appetite. Presumably this is because most or all of the reserve glucose (glycogen) is used up, and thus the blood glucose level will eventually decline. But the type of hunger produced by prolonged exercise is a different type of hunger. It's difficult to describe, but heavy exercise does not produce the sharp, almost trembling sensation of weakness that typifies the kind of hunger produced by inactivity (and a high sugar diet). Heavy exercise tends to produce a duller, much less intense hunger. The reason for this is not completely clear, but it probably relates to insulin regulation. It is well known that people who exercise tend to have much more stable insulin levels than people who do not exercise. Subsequently, people who exercise tend to have more even and stable blood glucose levels, and therefore would tend to experience more moderate hunger sensations.

In the beginning, most of us shouldn't worry about the hunger sensations produced by heavy exercise, because unless we are already exercising heavily, we should begin slowly . . . and light exercise tends to reduce appetite, not increase it. Moreover, it would be ill-advised to begin both a diet program and a heavy exercise program at the same time. Both should be started in moderation (see Chapter 8).

THIRD STEP - LOSING WEIGHT

Once we have eliminated sugar from the diet, we are ready to make some substantial progress in weight loss. Indeed, in the vast majority of cases, the elimination of sugar will have guaranteed that we are no longer gaining weight. To begin losing weight, then all we need do is eliminate a few calories. As mentioned earlier, one pound of fat is equal to about 3500 calories. To lose one pound a week, all we need do is eliminate about 500 Calories/day from what we would otherwise need to maintain our body-weight. Table 6-1, is the number of Calories required for people of different sizes and sex to maintain their weight.

TABLE 6-1. CALORIES REQUIRED FOR PEOPLE OF DIFFERENT SIZES AND SEX TO MAINTAIN THEIR WEIGHT. Source: National Research Council.

Category	Age (years)	Weight (lbs.)	Height (in.)	Average Energy Needed (with range) (Calories)	
Males	11-14	99	62	2700	2000-3700
	15-18	145	69	2800	2100-3900
	19-22	154	70	2900	2500-3300
	23-50	154	70	2700	2300-3100
	51-75	154	70	2400	2000-2800
	76+	154	70	2050	1650-2450
Females	11-14	101	62	2200	1500-3000
	15-18	120	64	2100	1200-3000
	19-22	120	64	2100	1700-2500
	23-50	120	64	2000	1600-2400
	51-75	120	64	1800	1400-2200
	76+	120	64	1600	1200-2000
Pregnancy				+300	
Lactation (Breast feeding)				+500	

Remember that calories can be reduced through exercise, as well as a reduction in diet. Table 6-2 is the amount of calories that are burned up per hour for a given exercise. Note that the amount of calories can be substantial. For example, an hour of jogging can be the equivalent of ⅓ to ½ of the calories required for all day!

TABLE 6-2. ENERGY EXPENDITURES FOR VARIOUS EXERCISES.

Bicycling 6 mph	240 cals.
Bicycling 12 mph	410 cals.
Cross country skiing per hour	700 cals.
Jogging 5½ mph	660 cals.
Jogging 7 mph	920 cals.
Jumping rope per hour	750 cals.
Running in place per hour	650 cals.
Running 10 mph	1,280 cals.
Swimming 25 yds/min. for an hr.	275 cals.
Swimming 50 yds/min. for an hr.	500 cals.
Tennis – singles per hour	400 cals.
Walking 2 mph	240 cals.
Walking 3 mph	320 cals.
Walking 4½ mph	440 cals.

Note: The calories spent in a particular activity vary in proportion to one's body weight. For example, for a 100-lb. person, reduce the calories by ⅓; for a 200-lb. person, multiply by 1⅓.

Source: Nat. Institute of Health Pub. No. 81-1677.

In respect to diet, with the elimination of sugar, calorie counting (if we are so inclined) can be reasonably accurate. If we like, we can calculate our daily meals to allow us to lose as much or as little weight as we desire. Again, maximum weight loss should not exceed more than 2 lbs. per week, unless under constant supervision by a physician.[3]

EDUCATED MEAL PLANNING

In planning a meal, the first consideration, of course, is the entree, the protein containing portion of the meal. Most adults need 3 to 4 ounces of high quality protein with each meal. That is, 3 to 4 ounces of meat, cheese, eggs, or milk (one cup of milk would equal one ounce of meat, cheese, or one egg).

In respect to dieting, it is important to realize that there are high and low fat sources of protein. Eggs, cheese,* and most sausages are high fat protein sources. These products typically contain as much or more fat as they do protein (see Table 6-3).

TABLE 6-3. RATIO OF PROTEIN TO FAT CONTAINED IN COMMON HIGH QUALITY PROTEIN FOODS.

Food	Ratio of Protein	to Fat
Beef, choice grade trimmed, lean (raw)	79%	21%
hamburger, lean (cooked	71	39
regular (cooked)	54	46
Cheese, cheddar & american	43	57
cottage (skim)	90	10
cottage (creamed)	76	24
Chicken, fryer (raw)	79	21
Eggs	52	48
Fish, ave. of all species (raw)	86	14
tuna, canned in oil (drained)	61	39
Pork, medium fat class, separable lean	65	35
Sausage, pork (cooked)	26	74
polish, bologna & frankfurters (all meat)	37	63
thuringer & salami	43	57
Turkey, all classes	77	23

Adapted from USDA Agric. Handbook #8, Composition of Foods. 1975.

If we are attempting to lose weight, then obviously we should select low-fat protein foods. As the reader is probably well aware, frying can substantially increase the fat content. In the case of fish, which is most often eaten fried, the frying process can double the amount of fat present (as can baking or broiling in butter).

After selecting the entree, some sort of vegetable should be selected. The primary reason for a vegetable is as a source of fiber (see pp. 132, & 116). Vegetables, of course, also contain vitamins and minerals (discussed in Chaps. 7, 17, & 18). Without getting into a lot of technical details, about ½ cup is usually adequate. If we care to eat more than that, there certainly isn't any problem either from a nutritional, or a dieting (weight loss) point of view.

*Excluding cottage cheese, which is low in fats.

If the vegetable is eaten in the form of a salad, bear in mind that many salad dressings are very high in vegetable oil. The newer buttermilk type of dressings, are typically much lower in fat.

After the protein and vegetable, the carbohydrate needs to be selected. This is where a lot of people make a mistake. Quite often, people will substitute another protein food or a larger portion of protein for the carbohydrate. As explained on p. 24, protein can be just as fattening as carbohydrate. Once the body's requirement for protein is met, any further protein will simply be broken down for use as energy.

In selecting a carbohydrate, try to select a complex carbohydrate. As explained earlier (p.14), complex carbohydrates take longer to digest, and thereby give us more opportunity to burn the calories off. Whole cereal grains, such as corn or hominy are excellent choices. Potatoes are also an excellent choice (baked or mashed — french fries, of course, contain substantial fat). If rice is on the menu, brown (unpolished) rice is best. The fibrous coating surrounding the starch in brown rice causes the starch to be digested much more slowly than polished rice (rice with the fiber removed).

The last choice should be white bread. Bread, or other products made with refined flour (or cornstarch) are digested much more quickly than whole grains, potatoes, or brown rice. As explained on p. 15, this is because the protective coating surrounding the starch has been removed. Thus, these products are called refined carbohydrates. (If we are going to be physically active shortly after eating, the type of carbohydrate is not as critical.)

The addition of fruit is often a good idea, particularly if fish is on the menu (see p. 114). Fruit, of course, adds vitamin C (potatoes also contain vitamin C), but fruit is also a good source of fiber and carbohydrate. If you are used to eating dessert, substituting fruit is a good idea.

In planning our meals, we can, of course, design them to fit a calorie budget. As mentioned earlier, once sugar is removed from the diet, calorie counting can be reasonably accurate. However, in the opinion of the author, it really isn't any fun to go through life eating our meals with a calculator. In the long run, a much more acceptable approach is to simply be aware of the approximate energy value of different foods and take that into account when deciding on a meal.

Table 6-4 categorizes most commonly eaten foods into equivalent calorie categories. If we select one item from each of the 4 different food group listings three times a day, there wouldn't be enough

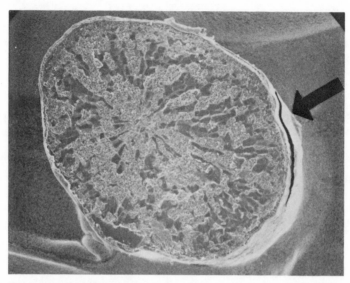

Figure 6-1a. Brown (unmilled) rice is covered with a tough, fibrous coating (see arrow), that slows down digestion of the starch contained within the rice grain itself. This outer coating (shown in closeup in Figure 6-1b), thereby causes the energy (calories) to be released somewhat slower than it would be if the coating were removed (as in milled or polished rice). For this reason, brown (unmilled) rice is usually less "fattening" than white (milled rice).

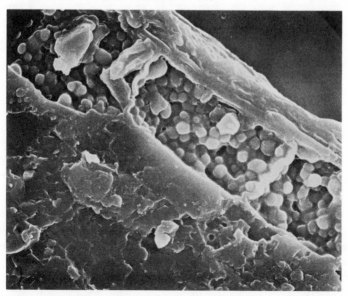

Figure 6-1b. Closeup of outer coating of unmilled rice. (Photos 6-1a & b courtesy of Cheryl Earp, Texas A&M Dept. of Grain Chemistry).

calories for a normal person to gain weight. Add to this 2 cups of milk, and the average caloric intake on a daily basis would be 1868 . . . about 200 less calories than most women need to maintain their bodyweight, and about 700 calories less than what most men need.

TABLE 6-4. EQUIVALENT CALORIE CATEGORIES OF COMMONLY EATEN FOODS.

Entree - Equivalents (Protein Foods)	Calories	Rate of Digestion
1 cup skimmed cottage cheese	125	moderate
3 ounces broiled lean beef, chicken (1 large breast) fish, or pork 1 cup creamed cottage cheese	135-150	moderately slow
3 ounces lean hamburger (10% fat), fried chicken (1 large breast) fried fish, roast pork, or roast turkey	160-185	moderately slow
3 eggs 4 ounces commercial hamburger (21% fat), cured ham, or fried shrimp, part skim cultured cheese (mozarella & ricotta)	235-275	moderately slow
Vegetables		
½ cup asparagus, broccoli, green beans, wax beans, beets, cabbage, carrots, cauliflower, lettuce, or summer squash	10-30	moderately slow
½ cup black-eyed peas, lima beans, or green beans	75-150	moderately slow
Carbohydrates		
1 cup most <u>unsweetened</u> whole grain dry cereal products (shredded wheat, etc.).	80-125	moderate
1 cup corn, brown rice, or hominy 1 ave. size potato or yam plus 1 Tbsp. sour cream	140-180	moderate
1 cup polished rice, 2 slices white bread, 1 cup spagetti pasta	140-180	moderately fast
Fruits		
1 apple, banana, or pear	100-125	moderate
1 orange or peach; 2 apricots, plums or tangerines; 1 cup bluberries, black-berries, cherries, grapes, raspberries, strawberries; ½ cantalope	40-80	moderate
1 avacado	300-400	moderately slow

This brings us back to the basic premise of this diet plan . . . that no one need cut back on basic food staples to afford weight control. Eating a diet such as this would allow anyone to control bodyweight without having to go around hungry in the process. That is, if we were to eat 4 ounces of meat, ½ cup of vegetables, a whole potato or a cup of corn or rice, and 2 or 3 apricots or a cup of berries at every meal, three times a day . . . I doubt seriously if any of us would walk away hungry.

Then, why do people gain weight? Very simple. Most people don't eat half a cup of vegetables, or a cup of rice, and a cup of fruit. They substitute other foods. Foods of greater caloric density.

Most people have never had the opportunity to realize just how potent sugar, corn starch, and flour are, as sources of food energy. They simply think of them as starches, just like potatoes and other carbohydrates. The fact of the matter is that one ounce of candy is the caloric equivalent of one whole potato! Most of us wouldn't even consider sitting down and consuming two large potatoes at a meal, but we think nothing of eating a piece of pie, which actually has a greater caloric value.

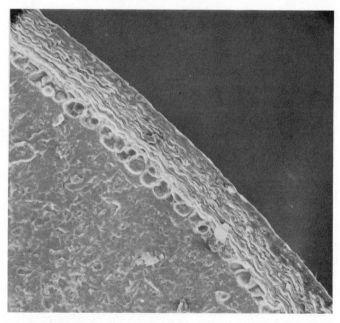

Figure 6-2. Cereal grains such as corn and wheat also have an outer layer of fiber that slows down digestion of the starch inside. Therefore whole cereal grains are less "fattening" than milled grains such as corn meal, flour, etc. (Photo courtesy Dr. Carl Hoseney, Kansas State University).

If you watch overweight people in cafeterias . . . they don't eat vegetables. They might eat salads (with ample dressing), but they do not eat vegetables. What they do eat is bread and rolls, crackers, fried foods, gravies, cobbler, puddings, and other desserts. Likewise you will usually find that they drink soda pop or other sugared beverages. All in all . . . very heavy on refined carbohydrates.

DIETING TIPS

Breakfast. We all know that breakfast is the most important meal of the day. However, the traditional bacon, eggs, and toast type breakfast is unnecessarily high in fat, refined carbohydrates, and almost devoid of fiber.

Eggs supply the same amount of fat as they do protein. Bacon and most sausages contain twice as much fat as protein. Toast, of course, is made almost entirely of refined carbohydrate (flour). Even whole wheat toast supplies very little effective fiber, since the whole wheat flour used in commerical bakeries is typically ground very fine.

If you like sausage (as I do), it is relatively easy to prepare a low fat product at home. All you need is some lean ground pork, sage, and black pepper. When eating in restaurants, of course, lean sausage is usually impossible to obtain. However, whenever traveling, I find that most restaurants will supply a small hamburger patty on request, even though it usually isn't listed on the breakfast menu. Commercial hamburger usually contains less than half as much fat as commercial sausage. An excellent breakfast can consist of a hamburger patty, some whole grain cereal (shredded wheat, etc.), and fresh fruit.

When eating at home, I have become fond of eating breakfasts that might ordinarily be considered lunch or dinner fare. A grilled pork chop, applesauce, hashbrowns, or a piece of roundsteak, fruit salad, and cottage potatoes not only hit the spot, but supplies the protein, carbohydrate, and fiber that we need.

On this subject, use your imagination. By reducing the fat and refined carbohydrate in your breakfasts, I think you'll also discover meals that can actually be tastier, and more satisfying.

Sour Cream vs. butter. Sour cream contains about ¼ as much butterfat as butter, and therefore has about ¼ as many calories. Obviously then, when dieting sour cream makes a better potato topping than butter. Likewise sour cream has about ¼ as many calories as margarine.

Salad dressings. As mentioned earlier, some salad dressings are extremely high in vegetable oil (fat). (Several commercially prepared varieties also contain sugar and other sweeteners.) Some of the newer buttermilk type dressings are much lower in fat (and calories).

Alcoholic beverages. Many people consider alcoholic beverages a part of their lifestyle and not part of their diet. As a result they are unwilling to consider reducing their intake.

There is no denying that alcohol is a major item in the lifestyle of many people. But there is also no denying that alcohol is a concentrated source of food energy. If we go to a party and consume three beers, or three glasses of wine, we may as well eat three large potatoes . . . its the same difference. We must understand that like sugar, alcohol is a potent and empty form of calories (see Chap. 9).

Read the label. As the reader is probably aware, sugar is used as a major ingredient in a large number of prepared food products. Although the popular press has done a good job of bringing these products to our attention, I think it worthwhile to review some of them.

An item that really had me fooled was prepared yogurt. Sold as "low fat" and advertised as a diet food, most commercially prepared yogurt is in fact a high calorie food. Yogurt by itself has a very acrid taste, and so fruit and a substantial amount of sugar is usually added. The end result is that most of the little 8 ounce cartons that appear to be ideal diet foods (high in protein, etc.), actually contain over 250 calories! This doesn't mean that yogurt itself isn't a good food, but it does mean that we need to read the label of the prepared products that we buy. If you like yogurt, you can buy (or culture yourself) unsweetened yogurt, and then add your own fruit.

Breakfast cereals are the items most often pointed out as being inordinately high in sugar . . . and indeed, many of them are. Because of this, there has been a serious discussion about introducing a bill before Congress to make it illegal to advertise these products during television programs aimed at children. The justification being that these products are little more than candy, but are used with the idea of providing nutrition (substituted for more nutritious foods).

Possibly as a result of the concern over the lack of nutrition in breakfast cereals, there are now a number of "high vitamin" cereals. Keep in mind that the addition of synthetic vitamins really doesn't make one cereal "better" than another one. As explained in chapter 7, a balanced diet supplies all the vitamins that a normal person requires.

As mentioned earlier, canned fruits are typically packed in sugar syrup. Fortunately, at the present time there are now products packed only in natural fruit juices (see Figure 6-4).

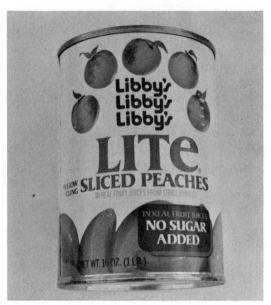

Figure 6-3. Read the label. Low sugar products are available, but it takes some looking.

The list of products that contain significant amounts of sugar is substantial: ketchup, canned meats, bullion mixes, spagetti and taco sauces, imitation dairy products, etc., etc., and on and on. Unbelievably, even some orange and grape juice products contain added sugar. The point of the discussion is simply to read the labels. Products without added sugar are available but it takes some examination to find them.

TYPES OF SUGAR

Rather than cut down on sugar, many people have turned to other types of sugars instead. In most cases the so-called natural sugars are essentially the same thing as table sugar.

Brown sugar. Brown sugar, often thought to be a raw or unrefined sugar is not that at all. It is actually white sugar that has had a trace of molasses added back to it. It is identical to white sugar.

Molasses. Molasses is, of course, a by-product of sugar refining. Although not quite as concentrated as white sugar, it is essentially the same thing.

Maple syrup. The sugar contained in maple syrup is identical to table sugar.

Honey. Honey contains the same componets as table sugar, but they are not totally bound together as in table sugar. That is, table sugar consists of two simple sugars bound together, glucose and fructose.

When glucose and fructose are bound together, they are known as sucrose (table sugar), which has a certain potential as a sweetner. When glucose and fructose are not bound together, they have separate and different sweetening potentials. Glucose is only mildly sweet, but fructose is intensly sweet. Fructose has approximately three times the sweetening potential of sucrose (table sugar).

Honey consists of both glucose and fructose, but only a very small percentage is bound together as sucrose. Because there is so much free fructose, honey is approximately twice as sweet as table sugar.

Whether it is "better" to use honey than table sugar is difficult to answer. From a dieting standpoint honey would yield fewer calories since less would be required for the same level of sweetness.

Purified fructose. Purified fructose products have become available in the last few years. As mentioned in the honey section, fructose has three times the sweetening power of table sugar. Therefore, for obtaining a certain level of sweetness, much less of these high fructose products are required. However, purified fructose has never been used to a large extent, and it is not known what the long term effects on the body might be.

PUTTING IT ALL TOGETHER

So far this chapter has discussed three basic principles concerning weight control:

1. The different type of calories in food (and the rate of digestion for each)
2. The amount of food eaten (or required)
3. Exercise programs

Putting all three of these principles together involves the concept of timing of intake. All this means is that we need to adjust the kind and amount of food we eat to coincide with our expected physical activity. Not only on a daily basis, but on an hourly basis.

If we want to eat sweets, then eat them just before exercising. In that way their fattening potential is greatly reduced or eliminated. Why? Because there is opportunity to burn up the energy they release, before it can be synthesized into fat.

If we're going to eat a set number of calories each day, spread them out evenly throughout the day . . . so that there isn't an excess of energy being released at any given time. For heaven sakes, don't follow the routine of eating a light breakfast and lunch, followed by a heavy dinner in the evening. Many of us have fallen into this trap, of course, because of family considerations. There is very little time in the morning and we cannot be with our families at lunch, so the evening meal takes on a sociological as well as a nutritional significance. As a result, the evening meal is usually much heartier than it should be. Obviously, going to bed on a full stomach is not the way to prevent fat synthesis from occurring. We should go to work, not to bed, on a full stomach. Adjusting our schedules to include a large breakfast and a light dinner in most instances requires a substantial change in lifestyle. The change is not only required of us, but of our families as well.

Keep in mind that this is where we originally came from. Before the urbanization of America, most families ate their large meal at noon. Indeed, among much of the farm population of the U.S. today, the noon meal is still called dinner, and the evening meal is called supper. Dinner is typically a hearty meal, and supper is a light meal (after the work is done).

For many of us, the advent of modern living has coerced us into changing our eating habits. Grandpa may talk about the rigors of having to go to work at the crack of dawn (down on the farm), but those of us who commute are no strangers to the pre-dawn hours. Getting up before daylight is not ordinarily conducive to a robust appetite.

Why did Grandpa feel like eating a large breakfast so early in the morning? Very simple. Because he went to bed early, and was able to sleep restfully. He was able to do this because he was physically tired.

If we try to go to bed early, we typically cannot sleep. Why?

Because we are not physically tired . . . we may feel tired, but we are emotionally tired, not physically tired. Grandpa worked with his back - we work with our minds. Grandpa had to work with mules - we have to deal with unreasonable people.

If we are to sleep, we must relax our minds, and tire our bodies. The only way to do this, of course, is to exercise. As explained in chapter 8, exercise can take our mind off our problems, and help us to sleep. Ultimately, we are able to awaken refreshed, and eat an appropriate breakfast. The end result is not only better weight control, but if we are better rested and nourished during working hours, the chances are that we will be more effective and successful in our employment as well.

But reducing the nutritional significance of our evening meal does not necessarily mean we have to reduce the sociological significance of our evenings. A family as a group can do more than just sit at the dinner table together. The entire family can be included in the exercise program. Tennis, softball, swimming, or just bicycling and jogging can be a family affair.

Certainly this type of change can be an abrupt modification in lifestyle. But like everything else in life, whatever is worthwhile obtaining, requires a commitment. In this case the commitment is capable of yielding not only a better physical appearance, but better health, and longer life. In addition, if we go to work better rested and with more energy, we may also be able to benefit financially as well.

In summary, it should be apparant that proper weight control is more than just a matter of dieting . . . it is a matter of education and lifestyle. It is not a matter of going on some sort of crash program every so often. It is a matter of understanding the basics of nutrition and health, and applying them to our daily lives.

Chapter 7 VITAMINS AND MINERALS
(WHAT WE NEED AND DON'T NEED)

At the present time there is a growing concern among health professionals in regards to what is termed "megavitamin and mineral therapy". Americans, at an increasing rate, are using vitamin and mineral supplements in excessive quantities. In some cases, the levels used are as high as 100 times the recommended allowances.

Short term massive doses of certain vitamins and minerals can result in symptoms of acute toxicity (which may include death). In most cases, the short term toxic effects of vitamins and minerals are well known. What isn't known, is what effect the long term taking of sub-toxic but otherwise excessive levels of vitamins and minerals may have. This is the reason for the concern.

In most cases, the taking of these compounds has not been undertaken because of advice from physicians or licensed dietitians. Rather, for the most part it has been prompted by articles appearing in popular magazines and books.

In some cases the public has been led to believe that massive doses of certain vitamins can cure otherwise incurable diseases. More commonly, people often question whether adequate levels of vitamins and minerals are obtained in the food they eat. Because of the high degree of processing, there is some question as to whether the vitamins are denatured and/or the minerals leached (washed) away. Less commonly, some people question whether the use of chemical fertilizers results in produce that has the same nutrient content as produce grown with organic fertilizers.

For the most part, the popular press has misled the public . . . the ideas about mystical properties of vitamins and minerals, and low levels in the food supply are unfounded.

At the present time, there are no known benefits to be obtained from vitamins or minerals, other than their metabolic roles. They can cure no diseases other than the metabolic diseases that occur when they are deficient. That is, there is nothing to be gained by taking massive doses. Vitamins have been said to cure everything from colds to cancer, but detailed research into these claims have shown them to be unfounded. That is, levels above the requirements have not been shown to have a positive pharmacological effect. Human nature being what it is, the idea of taking something that is said to be beneficial will often make us feel better whether it is effective or not. For that reason, in medical research, subjects are often given a placebo (sugar pill) while others are given the substance being tested. In many cases, persons receiving the placebo often report very favorable results. No doubt, the placebo phenomenon is responsible for much of the reported responses to vitamin supplements.

The idea that food grown with chemical fertilizers is any less nutritious than food grown with organic fertilizers is totally without foundation. Plants absorb nutrients in forms that are useful to them, and if the nutrients are not in those forms - they don't absorb them (and the plants don't grow). If a farmer wants to make a crop, his fertilizer has to have everything the plant requires. If it doesn't, he will get less than a maximum yield. Moreover, the idea that organically grown crops are more nutritious can be traced to health food retailers. Their motivation for making such claims is obvious, and their expertise in the area of plant physiology should be suspect.

The only area where the public's concern may be justified is in the area of food processing. The high degree of processing in some foods does reduce or eliminate the vitamin content, and in isolated incidences, the mineral content. For example, potatoes

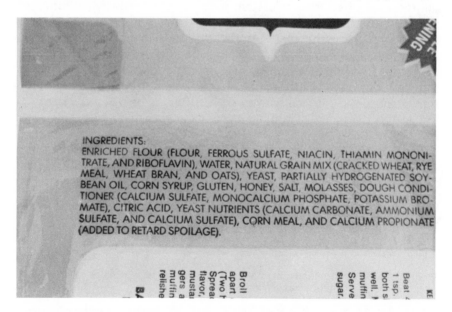

Figure 7-1. Most of the vitamins contained in wheat are removed during the milling process. However, B vitamins and iron are routinely added back to bakery products as "enriched flour".

are an excellent source of vitamin C, but commercially prepared instant mashed potatoes are practically devoid of vitamin C activity. Wheat and rice contain substantial levels of some of the B vitamins, but when the bran is removed (as in flour and polished rice), nearly all the B vitamins are removed as well.

Bear in mind, however, that nutritionists and food scientists are not unaware of this situation. For this reason, a great number of foods are enriched with vitamins and minerals. For example, several of the B vitamins plus iron are routinely added to flour and bread. One might question the wisdom of removing the vitamin containing portion of wheat (bran) in the first place (when the public could probably use the fiber), but the bottom line is that enough supplemental vitamins are used to make up the difference.

As a general rule, responsible health authorities and nutritionists are agreed that persons eating a balanced diet do not need additional vitamin or mineral supplements. The only exception to this would be pre-menapausal women and children who may need additional iron, and in some cases zinc.

Women may need additional iron because of menstrual losses and children because of growth requirements. Iron is a structural componet of hemoglobin and therefore anytime increased blood volume is required (menstruation, pregnancy, or growth), additional iron is required. Whether supplemental iron (and zinc) is required will depend upon the diet. If the diet is rich in meat, poultry, and/or fish, supplementation may not be necessary (except during pregnancy). Animal proteins are not only good sources of iron and zinc, but also greatly enhance the digestion of iron from vegetable sources. Typically iron absorption is increased about 3 fold in the presence of animal proteins (excluding dairy and egg products).[7]

With those exceptions it is generally agreed that vitamin/mineral supplements are not required by healthy persons eating a balanced diet. When deficiency diseases do occur, it is usually the result of some sort of metabolic problem or induced malnutrition.* The most common situation being alcoholism.**

Prior to the discovery of the existence of vitamins (and the

*Vegetarians need supplemental vitamin B12, since animal proteins are the only natural source. In addition, iron, and zinc are required.

**As explained in chapter 9, alcohol can reduce the absorption of several nutrients. A complicating factor is that alcohol often enhances the absorption of iron which is also high in some alcoholic beverages such as wine. Excess iron is toxic to the liver, which is a real consideration in alcoholism. Since most vitamin/mineral supplements contain iron - a special formulation is required.

need for a balanced diet), this was not the case. Probably the most classic example being the scurvy (vitamin C deficiency) that plagued European sailors in the middle ages. This was a major problem until the British Navy discovered that lime juice would eliminate the symptoms. From then on, limes were mandatory rations for British sailors, which earned them the nickname, "limeys".

At approximately the same time in history, Japanese sailors were plagued by beri-beri (vitamin B_1 deficiency). Later it was learned that the consumption of whole (brown) rice instead of polished (white) rice would eliminate the problem. But it was not until 1912, that the actual factor was isolated. An obscure scientist by the name of Cassimir Funk isolated the compound thiamine (vit. B_1). Funk then postulated the theory of minute compounds vital to life, and coined the term "vitamine". Vita for life, and amine because thiamine was an amine (nitrogen containing compound). When it was discovered that not all vitamins were amines, the "e" from vitamin was dropped.

In the U.S., the most classic example of vitamin deficiency was pellagra (niacin deficiency), which occurred with agonizing frequency among poor black sharecroppers and laborers in the South. Caused by the diet of corn meal, molasses, and salt pork they subsisted on, the disease was thought to possibly be due to an infectious agent caused by the wretched living conditions they endured. It was not until 1917, that the actual cause was identified. At that time a medical doctor by the name of Goldberger, working with the Public Health Service experimentally produced the disease in penitentiary inmates. The prisoners were told that they would be granted a pardon, if they would eat a corn meal based diet, instead of the usual prison food. Within 6 months, classic symptoms of pellagra appeared.

In the U.S. and other developed countries, whenever deficiency diseases have been identified, steps have been taken to prevent them. For example, vitamin D is required for the absorption of calcium and phosphorous. When cases of rickets appeared in children due to vitamin D deficiency, vitamin D was routinely added to milk. Milk was chosen because it is the richest source of calcium in the diet, which would insure that vitamin D would be there at the right time (see p. 145). When the cause of goiter was identified, iodine was routinely added to salt. When margarine began to displace butter on the dinner table, synthetic vitamin A was added to margarine.

The sum total of this being that deficiency diseases do not occur in healthy people eating a balanced diet. Most of the vitamins were isolated in the 1920's and 30's. The last one to be identified was in 1948 (vitamin B_{12}). Since that time there have been no new compounds discovered to be essential to life.*

THE RECOMMENDED DAILY ALLOWANCES (RDAs)

For the last 40 years the Food and Nutrition Board of the National Academy of Sciences has studied and evaluated the nutritional requirements for all nutrients, including vitamins and minerals. The results are published as the Recommended Daily Allowances (RDAs).[5] The RDAs are designed to "meet the known nutritional needs of practically all healthy persons". For that reason all the recommendations (with the exception of calories), are set high.** Even so, the scientists responsible for the RDAs have cautioned that this does not preclude the possibilty that the allowances may be too low for certain individuals. There is a large variation in nutrient requirements between individuals, and therefore the RDAs should not be considered as adequate for all persons.

Even with those limitations, it is useful to examine the vitamins and minerals contained in our diet. Table 7-1 is the RDAs for vitamins and minerals. Table 7-2 is the vitamins and minerals contained in a sample diet (as discussed in Chap. 6).

NOTES ON SAMPLE DIET

Vitamin A. The sample diet provided enough vit. A for women, but was slightly deficient for men. This really isn't of practical significance. Vitamin A is stored in the fat and liver and can be mobilized and used when the diet is deficient. There are some foods that are very high in vitamin A activity and when those foods are eaten the excess is stored for later use. For example, 1 cup of broccoli contains over 4000 units of vitamin A activity, and would supply the daily requirement by itself.

*In fairly recent times there have been some minerals isolated that were found to be nutritionally essential (nickel, silicon, vanadium, molybdenum, tin, etc.). However, the requirement is so small that it would be impossible to develop a deficiency without a synthetically produced purified diet. Indeed, the need for these minerals could not be proved until science was able to develop the very sophisticated techniques required for removing them from food. The need for these minerals is so infinitesimal, that as a practical matter they can be ignored.

**One of the primary difficulties in developing nutrient recommendations for humans lies in the type of research that can be done. In animal species, we can produce deficiency diseases, conduct growth study comparisons, and/or conduct life long metabolism studies. Obviously, these types of studies cannot be conducted with humans. As a result, the recommendations for humans are set high as a safety factor.

TABLE 7-1. RECOMMENDED DIETARY ALLOWANCES FOR VITAMINS AND MINERALS. (National Academy of Sciences)

	Age (years)	Weight kg	Weight lb	Height cm	Height in	Protein (g)	Fat-soluble vitamins Vitamin A (µg RE)†	Vitamin D (µg)‡	Vitamin E (mg α TE)§	Water-soluble vitamins Vitamin C (mg)	Thiamin (mg)	Riboflavin (mg)	Niacin (mg NE)‖	Vitamin B6 (mg)	Folacin¶ (µg)	Vitamin B12 (µg)	Minerals Calcium (mg)	Phosphorus (mg)	Magnesium (mg)	Iron (mg)	Zinc (mg)	Iodine (µg)
Infants	0.0-0.5	6	13	60	24	kg × 2.2	420	10	3	35	0.3	0.4	6	0.3	30	0.5**	360	240	50	10	3	40
	0.5-1.0	9	20	71	28	kg × 2.0	400	10	4	35	0.5	0.6	8	0.6	45	1.5	540	360	70	15	5	50
Children	1-3	13	29	90	35	23	400	10	5	45	0.7	0.8	9	0.9	100	2.0	800	800	150	15	10	70
	4-6	20	44	112	44	30	500	10	6	45	0.9	1.0	11	1.3	200	2.5	800	800	200	10	10	90
	7-10	28	62	132	52	34	700	10	7	45	1.2	1.4	16	1.6	300	3.0	800	800	250	10	10	120
Males	11-14	45	99	157	62	45	1000	10	8	50	1.4	1.6	18	1.8	400	3.0	1200	1200	350	18	15	150
	15-18	66	145	176	69	56	1000	10	10	60	1.4	1.7	18	2.0	400	3.0	1200	1200	400	18	15	150
	19-22	70	154	177	70	56	1000	7.5	10	60	1.5	1.7	19	2.2	400	3.0	800	800	350	10	15	150
	23-50	70	154	178	70	56	1000	5	10	60	1.4	1.6	18	2.2	400	3.0	800	800	350	10	15	150
	51+	70	154	178	70	56	1000	5	10	60	1.2	1.4	16	2.2	400	3.0	800	800	350	10	15	150
Females	11-14	46	101	157	62	46	800	10	8	50	1.1	1.3	15	1.8	400	3.0	1200	1200	300	18	15	150
	15-18	55	120	163	64	46	800	10	8	60	1.1	1.3	14	2.0	400	3.0	1200	1200	300	18	15	150
	19-22	55	120	163	64	44	800	7.5	8	60	1.1	1.3	14	2.0	400	3.0	800	800	300	18	15	150
	23-50	55	120	163	64	44	800	5	8	60	1.0	1.2	13	2.0	400	3.0	800	800	300	18	15	150
	51+	55	120	163	64	44	800	5	8	60	1.0	1.2	13	2.0	400	3.0	800	800	300	10	15	150
Pregnant						+30	+200	+5	+2	+20	+0.4	+0.3	+2	+0.6	+400	+1.0	+400	+400	+150	††	+5	+25
Lactating						+20	+400	+5	+3	+40	+0.5	+0.5	+5	+0.5	+100	+1.0	+400	+400	+150	††	+10	+50

* The allowances are intended to provide for individual variations among most normal persons as they live in the United States under usual environmental stresses. Diets should be based on a variety of common foods in order to provide other nutrients for which human requirements have been less well defined. See text for detailed discussion of allowances and of nutrients not tabulated. See Table (reverse page) for weights and heights by individual year of age.

† Retinol equivalents. 1 Retinol equivalent = 1 µg retinol or 6 µg βcarotene. See text for calculation of vitamin A activity of diets as retinol equivalents.

‡ As cholecalciferol. 10 µg cholecalciferol = 400 IU vitamin D

§ α tocopherol equivalents. 1 mg d-α-tocopherol = 1 α TE. See text for variation in allowances and calculation of vitamin E activity of the diet as α tocopherol equivalents.

‖ 1 NE (niacin equivalent) is equal to 1 mg of niacin or 60 mg of dietary tryptophan.

¶ The folacin allowances refer to dietary sources as determined by *Lactobacillus casei* assay after treatment with enzymes ("conjugases") to make polyglutamyl forms of the vitamin available to the test organism.

** The RDA for vitamin B₁₂ in infants is based on average concentration of the vitamin in human milk. The allowances after weaning are based on energy intake as recommended by the American Academy of Pediatrics) and consideration of other factors such as intestinal absorption; see text.

†† The increased requirement during pregnancy cannot be met by the iron content of habitual American diets nor by the existing iron stores of many women; therefore the use of 30-60 mg of supplemental iron is recommended. Iron needs during lactation are not substantially different from those of nonpregnant women, but continued supplementation of the mother for 2-3 months after parturition is advisable in order to replenish stores depleted by pregnancy.

TABLE 7-2. VITAMIN LEVELS CONTAINED IN A SAMPLE DIET.
(as recommended in chapter 6)

Food	Portion	Vit. A (I.U.s)	Vit. D (micrograms)	Vit. E (milligrams)	Vit. C (milligrams)	Thiamine (milligrams)	Niacin (milligrams)
Breakfast							
Pork (fresh, lean sausage)	2 ounces	0		.14	0	.63	3.8
Milk (whole)	1 cup	310*	100	.09	2	.09	.2
Shredded wheat	2 biscuits	0		.15	0	.12	2.2
Grapefruit	½	540			44	.05	.2
Orange juice	1 cup	500		.10	100	.17	.7
Snack							
Apple	1 whole	120		.46	6	.04	.1
Lunch							
Beef	3 ounces	10		.31	0	.05	3.6
Potato	1 whole	trace		.06	31	.15	2.7
Sour cream	1 tablespoon	90		.07	trace	trace	trace
Lettuce (salad)	1 cup shredded	180		.50	3	.03	.2
Salad dressing (soybean oil base)	2 tablespoons	50		7.37		trace	trace
Green beans	½ cup	340		.75	8	.05	.3
Milk	1 cup	310*	100	.09	2	.09	.2
Snack							
Orange	1 whole	260		.03	66	.13	.5
Dinner							
Chicken	4 ounces	50		.66		.03	2.7
Brown rice	1 cup	0		1.0		.23	2.1
Green peas	1 cup	1,170		.88	14	.15	1.4
		3,390	200	12.67	276	2.34	20.9

Vitamin D. Notice that the entire requirement of vit. D was contained in the two glasses of milk. When the skin is exposed to sunlight, the body can create its own vitamin D. The amount of time required depends upon the darkness of skin and the intensity of the sunlight. It is the ultraviolet rays that cause the vitamin to be formed, so one must be outdoors for sunlight to be effective (window glass filters out the ultraviolet rays).

Dark skinned peoples living in northern latitudes are most susceptible to vitamin D deficiencies. Dark skin pigmentation tends to block out penetration of the ultraviolet rays. In a tropical type of environment, of course, this is a definite advantage. In a more northerly environment, where sunlight may be limited (during the winter, etc.), it can result in reduced synthesis of vitamin D.

Because vitamin D deficiencies have occurred, vitamin D is routinely added to commercially processed milk (levels in unprocessed milk are quite variable). Vitamin D is added to milk so as to provide the adult requirement (200 units) in 2 glasses of milk. Vitamin D is required for calcium and phosphorous digestion, so milk was chosen as the best food to fortify.

Riboflavin (milligrams)	Vit. B$_6$ (milligrams)	Vit. B$_{12}$ (milligrams)	Calcium (milligrams)	Phosphorous (milligrams)	Potassium (milligrams)	Magnesium (milligrams)	Iron (milligrams)	Zinc (milligrams)
.09	.25	.9	7	181	192	11.0	2.2	2.5
.40	.10	.10	291	228	370	31.2	.1	.03
.06	.05	0	44	194	174	33.3	1.8	
.02	.03	0	20	20	166	29.0	.5	
.05	.03	0	25	45	496	20.5	1.0	
.03	.05	0	10	14	152	13.0	.4	
.14	.44	1.53	7	146	202	15.3	2.2	5.7
.07		0	14	101	782	28.0	1.1	.9
.02			14	10	17	2.0	trace	
.03		0	11	12	96	24.0	.3	
trace		0	2	3	18		.1	
.06	.05	0	32	23	95	25.0	.8	2.1
.40	.10	.10	291	228	370	31.2	.1	.03
.05	.06	0	54	26	263	14.0	.5	
.15	.50	.45	15	89	117	23.0	.9	1.9
.02	.18	0	21	57	57	46.0	1.8	2.0
.10	.16	0	44	129	163	60.0	3.2	.7
1.69	2.05	3.08	892	1,506	3,730	406	17.0	15.86

Babies and children kept indoors should be fed fortified (vit. D) milk. Mothers who nurse their babies should likewise consume fortified milk. If the mother is deficient in vitamin D, her milk will likewise be deficient.

If vitamin D supplements are used, be very careful with them. Vitamin D can be quite toxic at high levels (p. 145).

Folacin. Calculations for folacin were omitted due to a lack of standardized values for foods. Apparently folacin is difficult to analyze, and therefore printed values for foods vary substantially. Alcohol destroys folacin, and most deficiencies relate to alcoholism.

Calcium. Note that 65% of the calcium came from the two glasses of milk in the diet. Dairy products are essentially the only high calcium food in the human diet.

Most people recognize the requirement for calcium in bone growth, and therefore the need for children to drink milk. Unfortunately, many people do not realize that calcium is also a vital ingredient in muscle contraction. If the blood level of calcium drops too low, the body can go into tetany, and death can result.

To prevent this from happening, the body will pull calcium out of the bones for use in the blood and muscles. This, of course, weakens the bones. The medical term is osteomalacia, and it occurs with frequency in the elderly. The bottom line, is that dairy products are vitally important for adults as well as children.

Iron. As can be seen, the iron requirement was met for men, but was just shy for women. Inclusion of high iron foods such as raisins, or consumption of slightly more meat would bring the level up to the recommended levels. During pregnancy, women should probably take an iron supplement upon the advice of her physician. Likewise, nursing mothers should also probably take an iron supplement.

Iodine. The amount of iodine contributed by the diet was not calculated due to the highly variable levels found in foods. Plant foods will reflect the level found in the soil, and animal products are a reflection of the level found in their rations.

The National Research Council has determined that iodine consumption in the U.S. is adequate. In some cases, there is concern that it may be excessive. Iodate dough conditioners are sometimes used in breadmaking, which places enough iodine in the bread to meet the iodine requirement with one slice. Iodine disinfectants are sometimes used in dairies which increases the iodine content of dairy products.

Goiter, enlarged thyroid gland, is the deficiency symptom associated with insufficient iodine. While it used to be a common problem in the central U.S., the use of iodized salt has all but eliminated it.

However, it should be pointed out that much of the salt used in commercial preparation of foods is not iodated. Also, because salt consumption may be linked to hypertension (high blood pressure), it has been recommended that most people restrict their use of salt in cooking, and at the table (since commercially prepared foods contain adequate salt). In iodine deficient areas, this could conceivably result on inadequate intakes (if bread is not made with iodate dough conditioners).

CONCLUSIONS

From the preceding discussion, it should be clear that a balanced diet supplies all the vitamins and minerals (with the exception of iron) that a healthy person requires. However, there are people who acknowledge that they don't eat a balanced diet, and therefore take vitamin/mineral supplements to make up the difference. In this case, it should be emphatically pointed out that there is more to a balanced diet than just vitamins and minerals. As discussed in Chap. 5, a balanced diet is required for proper metabolism, and is essential to good weight control. In addition, there are indications that a balanced diet is protective of a number of degenerative diseases and disorders (Chap. 15 & 16).

If after careful consideration you deem it necessary to take a vitamin or mineral supplement, for heaven sakes be reasonable. Remember that there are no advantages to be gained from massive levels, but there are some very well known disadvantages. Aside from simple toxicities, high levels of most vitamins and minerals can tie up the absorption of other vitamins and minerals. Vitamins and minerals are relatively inexpensive to produce, and a higher level in one product does not make it better than another product. More is most definitely not better in vitamins and minerals.

If you decide to take a single vitamin or mineral supplement such as iron, take one that supplies only the level required to make up for what is missing in the diet. In some cases, the amount that the body actually absorbs may need to be taken into consideration. Your physician or a licensed dietitian are in the best position to advise you on that account.

If you take a multiple vitamin/mineral supplement . . . take a well balanced one. The Food and Drug Administration has set standards for products recommended for children, and pregnant or lactating women. Table 7-3 contains those standards. Unfortunately, there are a large number of products that don't fit those standards. Health food stores and even some pharmacies are filled with vitamin/mineral products that contain nonsensical combinations, or illogical levels. Typically these products are promoted as being a cure for some type of ailment or disease. Remember, if a product is effective as a treatment or preventative measure for a malady, it will say so on the label (see p. 4). The first ammendment allows a manufacturer, salesman, or retailer to make any claim about a product . . . he has the right to free speech. He can even print a totally untruthful piece of literature about the product. The FDA's labeling laws, however, forbid him from making an erroneous claim on the label of the product (see also Chap. 1).

	Unit of measurement	Children under 4 years of age†			Adults and children 4 or more years of age			Pregnant or lactating women		
		Lower limit	U.S. RDA	Upper limit	Lower limit	U.S. RDA	Upper limit	Lower limit	U.S. RDA	Upper limit
Vitamins										
Mandatory										
Vitamin A	IU	1250	2500	2500	2500	5000	5000	5000	8000	8000
Vitamin D	IU	200	400	400				400	400	400
Vitamin E	IU	5	10	15	15	30	45	30	30	60
Vitamin C	mg	20	40	60	30	60	90	60	60	120
Folic acid	mg	0.1	0.2	0.3	0.2	0.4	0.4	0.4	0.8	0.8
Thiamin	mg	0.35	0.70	1.05	0.75	1.50	2.25	1.50	1.70	3.00
Riboflavin	mg	0.4	0.8	1.2	0.8	1.7	2.6	1.7	2.0	3.4
Niacin	mg	4.5	9.0	13.5	10.0	20.0	30.0	20.0	20.0	40.0
Vitamin B_6	mg	0.35	0.70	1.05	1.00	2.00	3.00	2.00	2.50	4.00
Vitamin B_{12}	mg	1.5	3.0	4.5	3.0	6.0	9.0	6.0	8.0	12.0
Optional										
Vitamin D	IU				200	400	400			
Biotin	mg	0.075	0.150	0.225	0.150	0.300	0.450	0.300	0.300	0.600
Pantothenic acid	mg	2.5	5.0	7.5	5.0	10.0	15.0	10.0	10.0	20.0
Minerals										
Mandatory										
Calcium	g	0.125	0.800	1.200	0.125	1.000	1.500	0.125	1.300	2.000
Phosphorus	g	0.125	0.800	1.200	0.125	1.000	1.500			
Iodine	mg	35	70	105	75	150	225	150	150	300
Iron	mg	5	10	15	9	18	27	18	18	60
Magnesium	mg	40	200	300	100	400	600	100	450	800
Optional										
Phosphorus	g							0.125	1.300	2.000
Copper	mg	0.5	1.0	1.5	1.0	2.0	3.0	1.0	2.0	4.0
Zinc	mg	4.0	8.0	12.0	7.5	15.0	22.5	7.5	15.0	30.0

TABLE 7-3. VITAMIN AND MINERAL SUPPLEMENT STANDARDS FOR PREGNANT WOMEN AND CHILDREN. (Food and Drug Administration)

Chapter 8   EXERCISE - AN INTEGRAL PART OF ANY DIET/HEALTH PLAN

Exercise should be an integral part of any diet plan . . . not just to aid in weight loss, but to make us look healthy and attractive. With diet alone, we can lose weight, but we will not look or feel particularly healthy.

Those of us who have weight problems typically have sedentary type employment. During working hours we have very little opportunity for physical exertion. This, of course, is a tribute to our mental abilities and talents. But as intelligent creatures, we should not fail to take care of our body's requirements.

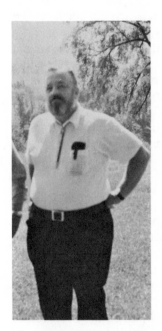
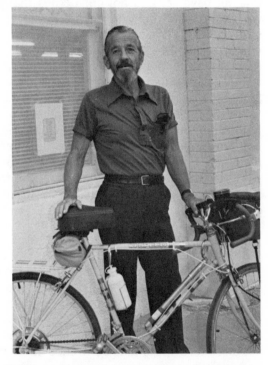

Figures 8-1a & 1b. Wayne Smith of Dalhart, TX at age 54 and 255 lb., and at age 56 and 152 lbs. The weight loss was a result of both dieting and exercise, and occurred within 9 months. As explained in chap. 6, that is actually more rapid than most physicians would recommend. Still, it demonstrates what self-determination can do. Wayne currently runs about 5 miles per day, and rides his bicycle about 12 miles per day. The bottom line (at age 58) is a blood pressure of 120/60 and a heart rate in the low fifties. (Photos courtesy of Wayne Smith, and Dalhart Texan Newspaper).

The problem is that sedentary occupations not only do not give us opportunity to exercise on the job, but can also tend to keep us from wanting to exercise at the end of the day. There are a number of reasons for this, but by far the most important is the amount of emotional stress that the majority of us must endure.

Emotional stress can make one feel physically exhausted. Financial problems, etc., can actually make us feel weak, and at times, even physically ill. Likewise, when we are forced to passively tolerate rude, obnoxious, or otherwise overbearing people, it is hard to get in the proper frame of mind for physical exercise.

We must realize, that it is the emotional strain of the day, not physical exertion, that is making us feel tired. In actuality, it is our psychic, and not our bodies that are tired. Physiologically we have a need to exercise. A need for exercise not only for the sake of our physical well-being (and appearance), but for our emotional well-being as well. Indeed, if we are to survive, we must be able to get our mind totally away from whatever it is that is causing us the stress.* Brisk physical exercise is the easiest and best way to accomplish this.

The first step toward getting in the proper frame of mind is to change our environment. It is amazing the difference that just putting on gym clothes will do. By putting on a pair of shorts, tee-shirt, tennis shoes, etc., we automatically begin to identify with physical activity. We tend to leave business problems, unreasonable or irrational people, etc., in the locker with our street clothes.

After changing clothes, go outside or to a gym where other people are working out. Ideally they should be people who take their exercise seriously. Their intensity is helpful in getting us to take our own exercise seriously. If you jog or work out with business associates, they should be friends whose kinship exceeds the confines of business related matters; people you can be yourself with.

By getting serious about our exercise program we not only exercise harder and thereby make more physical progress, but are also more apt to take our minds off of business related matters.**

*Being able to do this can mean the difference between having a heart attack, ulcer, or stroke at age 50, or continuing to be able to actively enjoy life through the retirement years.

**By being able to take our minds off of business, we are able to work more efficiently when we return. The mind is like everything else, it needs rest. When we are able to relax, solutions and creativity come more easily when we return to work. (There are, of course, people who would disagree with that . . . people who believe in "keeping your nose to the grindstone", 16 hours a day. Most typically, these are people who behave in a stereotyped manner, and seldom are capable of original thinking.)

EFFECT UPON THE HEART

Heart attacks, of course, are by far the leading cause of death. More importantly, heart attacks are the leading cause of premature death. The second leading cause of premature death is stroke. The chances of either one of these killers striking can be greatly reduced by daily physical exercise.

Quite obviously, exercise conditions the heart and vascular system to stress. By increasing the heart rate and blood flow, the arteries and veins are forced to expand and contract, and therefore become more resilient. This translates into lower blood pressure and a slower heart rate, which makes strokes and heart attack much less likely.

But even if a heart attack does occur, exercise greatly increases the likelihood of surviving the attack. Persons who exercise regularly are three time less likely to die during a heart attack.[6]

PHYSIOLOGICAL DIFFERENCES IN EXERCISES

Physiologically there are two different types of exercises; those that primarily condition the heart and lungs, and those that primarily build muscular strength and tone.

In order to condition the heart and lungs, the heart rate must be increased 60 to 75% its normal rate, and that rate must be held for at least 15 minutes. Table 8-1 lists average normal and conditioning heart rates for various age groups.

Exercises that do not increase the heart rate to at least 60% the normal rate for 15 minutes, will not afford much conditioning (will not be very protective against heart attacks).[6] Therefore, such activities as golf, bowling, volleyball, etc. do not really condition the heart. They can be beneficial by aiding coordination, eliminating stress, etc., but they do not substantially condition the cardiovascular system.

Studies by the National Institute of Health have determined that there is no real benefit to exceeding 75% the normal heart rate. Athletes in excellent physical shape can increase the heart rate to as much as 85% the normal rate, but that high a rate is no more protective than 75%.

Strength building exercises such as weight lifting, isometrics, etc. ordinarily do not condition the heart. Indeed, persons who have already had a heart attack or are otherwise prone to heart trouble should limit or avoid heavy strenuous type exercise or work. Heavy weight lifting, etc., increases blood pressure in relation to heart rate, by restricting the flow of blood back to the

TABLE 8-1. CONDITIONING HEART RATES DURING EXERCISE.

Age	Target Zone 60-75%	Average Maximum Heart Rate 100%
20 years	120-150 beats per min.	200
25 years	117-146 beats per min.	195
30 years	114-142 beats per min.	190
35 years	111-138 beats per min.	185
40 years	108-135 beats per min.	180
45 years	105-131 beats per min.	175
50 years	102-127 beats per min.	170
55 years	99-123 beats per min.	165
60 years	96-120 beats per min.	160
65 years	93-116 beats per min.	155
70 years	90-113 beats per min.	150

To find your target zone, look for the age category closest to your age and read the line across. For example, if you are 30, your target zone is 114 to 142 beats per minute. If you are 43, the closest age on the chart is 45; the target zone is 105 to 131 beats per minute. Your maximum heart rate is usually 220 minus your age. However, the above figures are averages and should be used as general guidelines.

Note: A few high blood pressure medicines lower the maximum heart rate and thus the target zone rate. If you have high blood pressure, obviously your physician should dictate what your target and maximum heart rate should be, as well as most other aspects of your exercise program.

Source: National Institute of Health Pub. 81-1677.

heart (during straining).[8]

HOW TO BEGIN AN EXERCISE PROGRAM

In the past, most authorities recommended that everyone consult a physician before commencing with an exercise program. At the present time, the National Institute of Health has taken a different view. The official position is that there are minimal risks for healthy persons to begin a gradual, sensible exercise program without prior consent of a physician. Quite obviously, there are some people who should consult a physician. Table 8-2 outlines people who should check with their doctor first:

TABLE 8-2. PERSONS WHO SHOULD CONSULT A DOCTOR BEFORE BEGINNING AN EXERCISE PROGRAM.

1. Over age 60, unaccustomed to exercising.

2. Have pains or pressure in the left or midchest area, left neck, shoulder, or arm — during or after exercise.

3. Have faint or dizzy spells.

4. Exertion leaves a state of extreme breathlessness.

5. Blood pressure is high.

6. Blood pressure is not known.

7. Have a family history of coronary artery disease.

8. Have elevated cholesterol or triglycerides.

9. Have had a heart attack, or other heart trouble (murmur, etc.).

10. Have any medical condition that might warrant special attention in an exercise program (insulin dependent diabetes, etc.).

Source: National Institute of Health Pub. 81-1677.

Reportedly there has been a lot of physician resistance to this type of approach. However, in the past it was felt that the old "see your doctor first", resulted in many people not exercising because they simply didn't want to go to the time and expense of having a physical.[9] As a matter of public policy, this new thinking is apparently based on the fact that exercise can literally save the lives of hundreds of thousands of people, while placing only a few individuals with unknown defects at increased risk.

SELECTING AND BEGINNING A BASIC PROGRAM

As mentioned earlier, there are two basic types of exercise programs; conditioning, and strength building. Everyone should at least adopt a conditioning program. Ambitious people may want to adopt a strength building program as well.

According to the National Heart Institute, to condition the heart and lungs one need only do conditioning exercises 3 times per week.[6] As explained previously, these exercises must raise the heart rate 60 to 75% for only 15 to 30 minutes. Further exercise will improve overall fitness, but 15 to 30 minutes is all that research has shown to be required to reduce the risk of heart problems. Jogging, bicycling, swimming, etc. will all accomplish this. Certainly it would seem reasonable to assume that increased fitness would add further protection . . . but apparently research has shown the maximum benefit/minimum effort relationship to be in this area.

Obviously, if someone is unaccustomed to exercise they should begin slowly. Before beginning jogging, vigorous calisthenics, etc., walking is an excellent exercise. It may take several weeks or even months before it is advisable to raise the heart rate 60% the normal rate. Common sense is the best guide.

Bear in mind that as fitness increases, the intensity of the exercise must increase to achieve the same exertion level. When first starting out, walking may increase the heart rate over 60%. As conditioning develops, a slow jogging will be required to obtain the same effect. Later, the jogging speed will have to be increased.

Once we have progressed to where we are able to do conditioning exercises 3 times a week at the required intensity level, we have a decision to make. Do we extend conditioning exercises to increase our endurance, or do we start a muscle tone or strength building program, or do we remain where we are. The decision, of course, is up to you. Most people, however, usually desire to progress once they have started an exercise program.

If the decision is to increase endurance, then all one need do is extend current exercise periods, or exercise more frequently. If the decision is to begin a muscle tone or strength building program, it may be accomplished by doing muscle developing or toning exercises one day, and conditioning exercises the next. If it is desired to conduct both exercise programs on the same day, maximum total benefit is usually accomplished by doing the muscle developing or toning exercises first. Do the muscle developing exercises while you have all your energy and strength, then burn up what's left over with 15 to 30 minutes of running, swimming, etc.

<u>Some notes on strength developing exercises.</u> Weight lifting
and isometrics are the most common strength building exercises.
However, certain types of gymnastic exercises and calisthenics
can also be good strength and tone builders.

As discussed on p. 63, only persons in good health should
begin a strength building exercise program. Lifting heavy weights,
prolonged straining, etc. increases blood pressure relative to
heart rate.

When beginning strength building exercises it is important
to begin slowly. As with all exercise, it is important to get the
heart, lungs, and circulatory system adapted to the increased
load. With strength exercises, it is also important to get the muscles
used to the extra load. Using too much weight or straining too
hard too quickly, will result in strained or even pulled muscles
and/or ligaments.

Also, when doing strength exercises it is important to be warm.
Working out in a cold room, etc. further increases the potential
for strained muscles. Likewise one should always "warm up"
before doing any muscular straining.

INDIVIDUAL EXERCISE PROGRAMS

The purpose of this chapter has not been to provide step by
step exercise courses. There are volumes of material available
on that. Rather, the purpose of this chapter has been to provide
information on the basics and the necessity of exercise. There
are any number of exercise programs that can be of benefit. The
program that appeals to the individual tastes of the reader, is
the one that he or she will be most likely to stick with . . . and
therefore will be the most beneficial. Whether the program be
calisthenics, jogging, basketball, bicycling, swimming, handball,
tennis, or any other vigorous activity . . . it makes no real difference. The crucially important thing is simply that a program
be selected, and adhered to.

Summary and final thoughts. In today's world it has become
fashionable to speak of sedentary type employment in a demeaning
manner. Outdoor/physically active occupations are often depicted
romantically, whereas indoor/office related occupations are often
depicted disdainfully. This, of course, is a warped sense of reality.
In order to maximize our contribution to society, we must seek
employment to our fullest capabilities. In most cases that means

we must work with our brains, rather than our backs. While yielding a net benefit to society, our contribution yields a detriment to us personally. A detriment in the form of reduced opportunity for exercise . . . and because of psychological stress . . . a reduced desire for exercise.

As intelligent persons we must not let this happen. We must realize that in spite of our intellectual powers, we are still biological creatures. If we are to prevent premature death, or otherwise ensure good health, we must compensate.

Aside from improved overall health and vitality, exercise also provides the side benefit of enhanced personal attractiveness (see Chap. 4). Unlike some forms of vanity, the personal appearance benefits of exercise is not mere self-indulgence. Instead of simply becoming more attractive, exercise makes us of greater value to society as a whole. By being physically fit, we typically are mentally more alert, and therefore able to work harder and in a more creative manner. In addition, should we ever encounter a situation calling on us to aid someone in physical distress, we would obviously be in a much better position to respond. Indeed, in the opinion of the author, this last thought is a very profound one. To watch a child drowning, or an elderly person trapped in a fire or attacked by a hoodlum, and to be unable to respond purely due to physical reasons . . . would leave a very deep psychological scar.

Chapter 9   ALCOHOL* IN THE DIET

In respect to dieting, it should be remembered that alcoholic beverages have nutritive significance as they add energy (calories) to the diet.   Indeed, many dieters tend to overlook the amount of energy alcohol can add (see p. 41).

In respect to nutrition and health, alcohol should not be thought of as a nutrient, so much as it should be thought of as a drug. Although many alcoholic beverages contain B vitamins and some trace minerals, with one exception, their significance is minimal since alcohol tends to interfere with absorption of most vitamins and minerals. For the most part, alcohol supplies what is commonly termed "empty calories".   It supplies no nutrients other than calories. The one exception to that is iron.

Although it is not clearly understood, alcohol tends to increase iron absorption.[10]   Ordinarily, something that increases iron absorption would be considered good, except in this case it can be potentially harmful since excessive iron can be toxic to the liver. Alcohol, of course, tends to damage the liver itself, and when it is considered that many alcoholic beverages, such as wine, contain relatively high levels of iron, the potential for liver damage is increased.   Of particular importance is the fact that alcohol tends to reduce the absorption of other vitamins and minerals. Thus, if a typical vitamin/mineral supplement is taken to compensate, liver damage may be even more accentuated since most vitamin/mineral capsules are heavily fortified with iron.

Calories added to the diet. By laboratory analysis, alcohol is much more fattening than carbohydrate. Alcohol contains about 7 Calories per gram, whereas carbohydrate only contains about 4. However, as pointed out in chap. 3, caloric values as determined by laboratory analysis, can be misleading. In actuality, alcohol does not seem to support the same amount of weight gain as its energy content would indicate.[11] Apparently this is due to the fact that alcohol increases heat production within the body. This, of course, is why alcohol tends to give one the feeling of warmth. The increased heat production increases the need for oxygen (creates heavier breathing), which is why alcoholic beverages decrease physical stamina.

---

*The term alcohol refers to ethyl alcohol (ethanol), commonly referred to as beverage alcohol. Methyl alcohol (methanol), of course, used in rubbing alcohol, disinfectants, etc. is a deadly poison.

Because of increased heat production within the body, alcoholic beverages obviously tend to make one more susceptible to environmental heat stress. Conversely, during cold weather when the increased heat production would seemingly be an advantage, in reality consuming alcoholic beverages can actually make one much more susceptible to hypothermia (loss of body heat resulting in death). This is because alcohol tends to open the capillaries near the skin's surface. During cold stress, the body's normal reaction is to close the capillaries and greatly reduce blood flow near the surface of the skin. The majority of the blood is kept near the core of the body (heart, lungs, etc.) in order to insulate the vital organs and conserve body heat. Circulating blood near the skin's surface greatly increases heat loss, even though the person actually feels much warmer than they would otherwise (without consuming alcohol). <u>It is therefore very ill-advised to give alcoholic beverages to anyone exposed to either heat or cold stress.</u>

Changes in the digestive tract. When alcohol use is extended over a long period of time, a number of physiological and enzymatic changes may occur in the digestive organs.

The first organ alcohol comes in contact with is the stomach. The walls of the stomach are lined with a mucous membrane, which is there to protect it from the intensely concentrated acid that is secreted to break down food. Alcohol tends to dissolve the mucus, thereby exposing the stomach wall to the action of the acid. The result is what is termed gastritis (severe burning sensation in the stomach). It is postulated that alcohol can be instrumental in the formation of stomach ulcers (by dissolving the mucus and allowing the stomach to be "digested" by its own acids and enzymes).

The effects on the rest of the digestive tract are many and varied. First of all, the upper end of the small intestine which the stomach empties into, also has a mucosal lining (to protect it from the still highly acid stomach contents). Alcohol tends to dissolve this mucus as well, and lesions are common when alcohol consumption is chronic.

Alcohol tends to interfere with the proper functioning of digestive enzymes found in the small intestine. Abnormal secretions of the pancreas and gall bladder often occur. Pancreatitis, a disease of the pancreas has been implicated in chronic alcoholism.[10]

Probably the most well known effects of alcohol are upon the liver. Among the many functions of the liver are the regulation of fat and cholesterol metabolism. As explained on p. 106, alcohol tends to greatly increase fat production. Continued alcohol consumption often causes much of this fat to be deposited around the liver, creating what is known as the "fatty liver syndrome". In addition to fat being deposited at the liver, much of it may be released to the bloodstream, thereby increasing blood triglycerides and (to a lesser extent) cholesterol levels. It is possible that this may be a factor in coronary disease.

With severe alcohol abuse, cirrhosis of the liver may occur. When this happens, a number of devastating physiological changes can take place. The liver's function of protein synthesis is greatly impaired, and therefore muscular emaciation is often a symptom. Another function of the liver is the conjugation of hormones, and therefore during acute cirrhosis, testicular degeneration and lack of libido (sex drive) sometimes occurs. The ability of the liver to filter toxic compounds out of the blood is impaired. As the reader is most certainly aware, cirrhosis is a life threatening situation.

SUMMARY AND CONCLUSIONS

Alcohol is a very high energy compound that is often overlooked by dieters as a significant source of calories. Alcohol alters body metabolism, and therefore its caloric value is not utilized as effectively as carbohydrates or fats. Still, it has substantial energy value, and can be very fattening when not taken into consideration. It apparently causes the liver to over-synthesize fats and fail to regulate cholesterol metabolism. As a result, blood triglycerides and cholesterol are often increased.

Chronic consumption of alcohol can tend to alter digestive organs and their functions. Symptoms may include gastritis, ulcers, dysfunction of the pancreas, and fatty liver. Severe alcohol abuse can ultimately lead to liver cirrhosis.

SECTION II - DIET, NUTRITION, AND HEALTH

Chapter 10 NUTRITION AND RESISTANCE TO INFECTIOUS DISEASES

Research studies with animals have shown that proper nutrition plays a major role in resistance to infectious diseases.[12] Observations with malnourished people have indicated the same thing.[13,14]

Infectious agents. The two basic types of organisms that cause a majority of the diseases that affect humans are bacteria, and viruses. It is vitally important to understand that bacteria and viruses are two totally different kinds of organisms.

Viruses are infinitely smaller than bacteria . . . so small that they cannot even be seen with a microscope (figure 10-1). The only way that viruses can be seen is with what is known as an electron micrograph. This is a piece of equipment developed only relatively recently, that can actually photograph individual molecules.

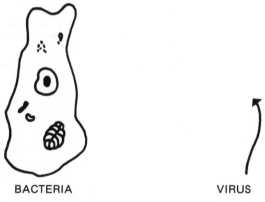

BACTERIA   VIRUS

Figure 10-1. Bacteria compared to virus (as seen through a microscope). Virus are so small, they cannot even be seen with a microscope.

Because bacteria can be seen with a microscope, scientists have known about them for a long time. Louis Pasteur, one of the first great microbiologists, identified the organisms that cause pneumonia in the 1850's. Indeed, pasteurella bacteria, the organisms that cause pneumonia, were named after Dr. Pasteur.

Antibiotics. Because scientists have known about bacteria and their role in disease for a long time, much effort was expended in trying to develop medicines to combat them. It was known that alcohol and other disinfectants would kill them on environmental surfaces, but what was needed was a drug that would function inside the body.

Early in this century penicillin was discovered. Effective against a broad range of bacteria, penicillin was heralded as a "wonder drug". Indeed, penicillin is effective against the organisms that cause pneumonia and tuberculosis. Overnight its discovery removed these two diseases as the number one and number two causes of death in the nation (Figure 10-2 & 10-3).

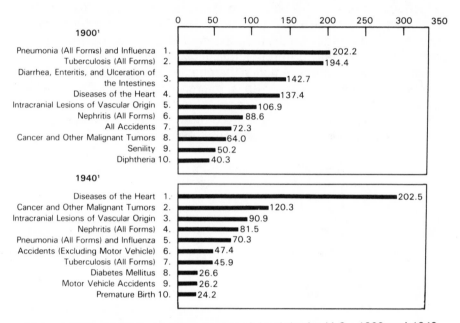

Figures 10-2 and 10-3. Leading causes of death in the U.S.; 1900 and 1940. The advent of penicillin dropped the pneumonia and tuberculosis death rate to ⅓ and ¼ of their previous rates. From National Institute of Health Pub. No. 81-2105.

Penicillin, of course, is one of a number of antibiotics which have been found to be effective in combating bacterial diseases. They function by attacking the vital organs (organelles) of the bacteria. In some cases antibiotics interfere with the nucleus which contains the genetic material. This keeps the bacteria from reproducing. In other cases, antibiotics function against the organelles responsible for digesting food or releasing energy. In other cases, antibiotics break open the cell wall that holds the bacteria together, and literally spills their guts out (Figure 10-4).

Controlling viral diseases. At this point it is vitally important to remember that viruses are totally different from bacteria. They

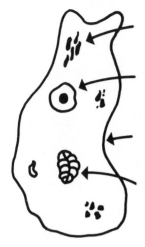

Lysosomes. The center for protein digestion. Some antibiotics kill bacteria by keeping them from digesting proteins.

Nucleus. The center of reproductive activity. Some antibiotics interfere with the genetic material and keep the bacteria from reproducing.

The cell wall. Many broad spectrum antibiotics break (lyse) the cell wall which literally spills their guts out.

Mitochondria. The center for energy metabolism. Some antibiotics "starve" the bacteria to death by interfering with the mitochondria.

Figure 10-4. Antibiotics function by attacking the organs (organelles) of bacteria. Viruses don't have organs like bacteria, and are immune to the action of antibiotics.

do not have organelles like bacteria, nor do they function like bacteria. For that reason, antibiotics are ineffective against viruses. If the reader gets nothing more out of this chapter, it should be that <u>antibiotics are ineffective against viral diseases.</u> This is one of the most basic, but least understood aspects in all of human or veterinary medicine.

The only way the body can protect itself against a viral infection is through its own immunity (defense) system. One of the primary agents in the immunity system is what is known as the antibodies.

Antibodies are agents formed within the body for destruction of foreign proteins. When a foreign protein such as a virus enters the body, antibodies are formed specifically for that particular protein. Somehow, the antibody recognizes the chemical make-up of the invading protein it has been formed to eliminate, and attacks it.

This is the idea behind vaccination. Vaccine is actually a weakened or killed form of a disease-causing organism. Thus, when someone is vaccinated against a particular disease, what occurs is that a killed or weakened form of the virus (or bacteria) is introduced into the body. The body then forms antibodies to attack the invading organism (vaccine). Hopefully, when naturally occuring virulent forms of the organism attack the body, antibodies will have already been formed. Thus, they will be able to destroy the invading organism before it is able to cause sickness.

FACTORS AFFECTING THE ABILITY TO PRODUCE ANTIBODIES

There are a number of factors that can affect the ability of the body to form antibodies. Anything that stresses the body can affect immunity. Lack of sleep, or becoming chilled are two prime factors. Observations with livestock have shown that even emotional stress can increase susceptibility to disease.

Nutrition can be a major factor in the ability to form antibodies. Since antibodies are comprised primarily of protein, protein deficiencies can obviously reduce antibody synthesis. Studies with animals fed low protein diets have demonstrated an increased susceptibility to disease.[13] In humans, malnutrition has generally been associated with decreased immunity. However, recent observations with young girls affected with what is known as "anorexia nervosa", have shown that decreased immunity does not occur until extreme emaciation occurs.[15]

Anorexia nervosa is a psychological problem in which young girls develop a neurotic fear of gaining weight. They therefore starve themselves into unnecessary and excessive weight loss. The starvation is different than other malnutrition, as when some food is eaten, it is usually a protein food. Also, vitamin/mineral supplements are often taken. As a result, energy is often the only nutrient in deficiency. From observation, it would therefore appear that in general protein/calorie malnutrition, it is the lack of protein that is directly responsible for reduction in immunity.

Vitamins and minerals. Deficiencies of individual vitamins and minerals can affect the ability to form antibodies. It has been reported that deficiencies of vit. A, several of the B vitamins, C, E, iron, and zinc can reduce the immune response.[16]

Probably equally important in this day and time, is the fact that excesses of certain vitamins and minerals can reduce immunity. Excesses of vitamin E, iron and zinc have been reported to decrease immunity. Given the large number of people who consume megadoses of vitamin E, excess vitamins and minerals can have clinical importance. As a result of a workshop on nutrition and immunity, the American Medical Association has recommended to its members to discern whether patients with immunological problems are consuming large doses of vitamins or minerals.[16]

FIGHTING COLDS, FLU, AND OTHER VIRUS DISEASES

From the previous discussion it should be remembered that

antibiotics are not effective against viruses. <u>At the present time, there is no medication that can be taken to combat viruses.</u> The only thing that can eliminate a virus is the immunological system of the body. In the case of colds and flu, there are a number of drugs that can be taken to reduce the effect of the symptoms . . . but there is nothing that can be taken to eliminate the virus itself. Only the body's immune defense system can do that.

As mentioned in the previous section, with many virus diseases, vaccines can be given to create an antibody level prior to infection with the disease. Also, with many diseases, once there has been an infection, the body will continue to produce antibodies so that the disease never occurs again. Cold and flu viruses, however, are apparently able to change their outer protein coating so that pre-formed antibodies cannot detect them. This is apparently the reason people can contract colds and flu so many different times. [17]

Since the immune system is the only defense against colds and flu, one should take extra precaution to get enough rest, and a balanced diet while ill. Numerous research trials have shown that massive doses of vitamin C are not effective in reducing the duration of illness. [18] Other studies, however, have shown a moderate increase in the requirements for vitamin A, C, and E during infection. [16] If it is desired to take additional vitamins, a balanced vitamin supplement (as discussed on p. 55), would be infinitely better than massive doses of a single vitamin. A balanced supplement would supply the moderate excess of vitamins A, C, and E which may be beneficial, would avoid extreme excesses of vit. E which can be detrimental, and assure adequate levels of several of the B vitamins, which can be detrimental when deficient.

In severe cases of colds and flu, doctors will sometimes prescribe antibiotics. When this is done, it is usually to reduce the likelihood of a secondary bacterial pneumonia from occurring. Unfortunately, many people believe that the antibiotics are effective against the cold and flu virus itself. This, of course, is not true. These people often think that by "getting a shot", they can function as though they are not ill; that is, not "take care of themselves". This is most certainly not true. Without adequate rest, proper nutrition, etc., the viral infection will continue for a longer period, and will probably be more serious. Again, there is no drug that can be taken to combat virus diseases.

Interferon. The compound interferon, which has made the headlines as a possible cure for cancer, may be our first opportunity to have an anti-viral drug. Interferon is actually produced in body cells, for combating virus that invade the inside of the cell. Interferon is part of what is known as the cellular defense system. That is, once virus actually enter the body's cells, they are beyond the reach of antibodies. Therefore, the body has a separate immune system for battling viruses inside the cells. In essence, the body has two different defense systems; the circulatory system, in which antibodies are the main component; and the cellular defense system, in which interferon is apparently a major component. Virus circulating in the blood and lymph system are attacked by antibodies, but once they enter the cells they are neutralized by interferon.

What makes interferon particularly valuable as an anti-viral drug is that it is non-specific. That is, it will neutralize nearly all types of viruses. This is very important since antibodies are specific for each kind of virus, and it typically takes 10 days to 2 weeks to form enough antibodies to effectively fight most serious viral infections.

What makes the development and production of interferon difficult is that it is host specific. That is, each species of animal has its own form of interferon, which will not function in another species. That eliminates the possibility of extracting it from animals for use in humans. (For example, insulin is extracted from the pancreas of slaughtered cattle, for use in humans.) At the present time, the only way interferon can be obtained is by extracting it from human white blood cells. The amount of interferon obtained this way is exceedingly small, and as a result the cost is astronomically high. Because of the cost, the experimental use of interferon has been primarily restricted to cancer, as cancer patients are willing to pay the necessary $1,500-2,000 per treatment. (Interferon apparently has anti-tumor properties as well as anti-viral capabilities.[19])

Currently there is much research being conducted into the possibility of producing interferon through what has come to be known as genetic engineering. Known to scientists as DNA recombinant research, the idea is to implant the genes of one species of life into another species. In this instance, the effort is being made to take the gene for interferon production from human cells, and implant it in a bacteria. Bacteria are cells similar to body cells, and are often attacked by virus. They therefore secrete a type of interferon. If scientists are successful in removing the bacterial gene for interferon, and replacing it with a human gene for interferon . . . the amount of interferon produced could be increased by billions of times the current level. That is, once a strain of bacteria capable of producing human interferon is developed, they could be reproduced and grown in whatever quantity is desired. The cost of interferon could be reduced to a few cents per treatment, rather than the current cost of thousands of dollars.

SUMMARY

The body has two different types of defense systems for preventing or overcoming infections. The first line of defense is the circulatory (humoral) system of which antibodies are the major component. The second line of defense is known as the cellular immunity system. Interferon, a compound produced in the cells is a major component of the cellular immunity system.

Antibiotics, commonly used to combat bacterial diseases, are not effective against viruses. The only agents that can eliminate viruses are the body's own immune defense mechanisms. Because nutrition and stress can reduce the ability of the immune response system to respond to infections, one must "take care of himself" when ill. Likewise, poor nutrition, becoming overtired (lack of sleep, etc.), chilled, or otherwise stressed can increase the chance of "catching" an infectious disease.

Chapter 11 DIET AND HYPERACTIVITY IN CHILDREN

This chapter is quite short, due to the fact that there is very little known about hyperactivity. A number of people have opinions (including the author), and those opinions will be expressed here (including the author's).

The condition. Professional psychologists and psychiatrists have identified a syndrome known as hyperkinesis or hyperactivity, in which children display reduced attention spans, appear to be constantly physically active, and reportedly have difficulty controlling their own behavior. Although children are often inaccurately diagnosed as being hyperactive (by non-professionals), a goodly number of children are believed to indeed be inflicted by hyperkinesis.

The cause or causes are unknown. In many cases, physicians have prescribed behavior altering drugs. Quite obviously, the continued use of drugs in young children has been a worry and concern to many parents.[20] It is not understood how the drugs work, and it appears that they may stunt growth.[21] The usual method has been to administer the drugs during the school year, and withhold them during the summer.

THE FOOD ADDITIVE-FREE DIET

In the mid 1970's a popular book was published by a pediatrician in which hyperactivity was said to be caused by substances found in food.[22] Food additives in general were said to be involved. In addition, naturally occurring compounds known as salicylates were also said to be involved (aspirin is a form of salicylate).

The book recommended that hyperactive children be put on a diet that excluded all synthetic food additives; no artificial colors, flavors, or preservatives. In addition, fruits and vegetables believed to contain salicylates were to be excluded; oranges, blackberries, grapes, raisins, currants, peaches, strawberries, tomatoes, and cucumbers were all to be excluded from the diet.

The book received widespread attention and publicity both in the popular and scientific press. Parents began putting their children on the recommended diet, and scientists began investigating the diet. The results have created controversy.

At the time the book was written, there was little information available on the amount of salicylates contained in foods. Laboratory assays done in response to the book, showed salicylates to be contained in practically all foods. Some of the foods that were included in the diet were actually higher in salicylates than those that were excluded.[23]   In a more recent publication, the role of salicylates has been reduced. The primary emphasis is now on artificial additives.[24]

Scientific evaluation. Scientific trials with the diet plan have produced confusing results.   These were trials in which children were split into groups and some of them received foods containing additives and others did not.   Some of the trials switched the diets so that children were exposed to both different diet treatments.

The primary problem with these diets was disguising them from the children and their parents.   In many cases parents were able to determine which diet their child was on, and this knowledge could have influenced their thinking (rating their child's behavior). That is, the placebo (sugar pill) effect is well known in science and medicine.   When people think something is beneficial, they often report a benefit, even if the medicine/drug is ineffective.

Reviews of these trials have reported that eliminating artificial food additives may reduce hyperactivity in a small percentage of the children tested. [21,25]

Opinion of physicians and scientists.   In general, the scientific community has a very reserved opinion.   In some studies, it does appear that certain food colorings may affect the behavior of a small percentage of children.   Unrelated studies with the flavor enhancer, monosodium glutamate, have shown that it can trigger a marked reaction in some people.   However, the reaction (commonly known as the Chinese Restaurant Syndrome) is more of an allergic type reaction, than a behavior modification.

Most health professionals see no physical problem with using the diet, as long as parents see to it that the child obtains enough vitamin C.   The diet restricts many of the more common sources of vitamin C, and therefore parents should see to it that the child consumes alternate sources (oranges are excluded, but not grapefruit, lemons, or limes).

Many health professionals are of the opinion that parents often have high hopes for the diet plan.   They feel that in some cases the positive expectations may tend to influence the parents' perception of their child's behavior in response to the diet.   "Since the plan does no physical harm, it might be helpful therapy due to its impact on the family".[23]   However, it has also been pointed out that there might be a negative effect . . . teaching the child (and his parents) to blame food ingredients on his behavior, when actual causes may be something totally different. [23]

OTHER THEORIES

Megavitamin treatment. There are some parents who have attempted to treat their children with high levels of selected vitamins; the thinking being that hyperactivity is a result of a vitamin deficiency.

Several well controlled studies have examined popular high level vitamin combinations. In these trials, children were split into groups and either fed high level vitamin supplements or a placebo (sugar pill, capsule filled with milk powder, etc.). In a review of these trials, it has been reported that behavior was often reported to be improved . . . but the placebo groups had as many or more responders as the high vitamin group. In one study using children who were also receiving behavior modifying drugs, two children were improved to the point that drugs were no longer deemed necessary. These two children were in the placebo group.[21]

Sugar. Popular magazines and books have often indicated sugar as a contributory factor. Relating stories of children "crawling the walls" after Halloween, many parents sincerely believe foods with a high sugar content cause a deterioration in their children's behavior.

The scientific community, for the most part, has remained skeptical. Stories by school officials, parents, etc., are often dismissed as being anecdotal. The typical opinion expressed is that sugar is simply a carbohydrate, and has no pharmacological properties.

COMMON SENSE CONCLUSIONS (Author's Opinion)

Certainly it is true that some individuals can have higher vitamin requirements than others. Indeed, the National Research Council points this out, and states that their recommended allowances may not be adequate for everyone.[5] However, the idea that vitamin deficiencies may be responsible for hyperactivity is illogical. That is not the way vitamin deficiencies work. When vitamins are deficient, their effect on behavior is that of lethargy, or anemia . . . not increased activity.

In certain cases, excesses of vitamins can produce toxicities that affect behavior. For example, vitamin A toxicity increases cerebro-spinal fluid pressure, which in animals has been known to cause hyperirritable aggressive behavior (large animals become dangerous). Quite obviously, megadoses of vitamins would tend to cause toxicities, and could therefore be considered a theoretically possible cause, not a cure, for hyperactivity.

In addition to being illogical, megadoses of vitamins can be quite dangerous. The short run toxic effects are quite well known. What is not known, are the long run effects of excessively high (but sub-toxic) levels of vitamins given over a long period of time. Quite clearly, to begin giving a child excessive doses of vitamins in his or her formative years, is an irresponsible act.

In the case of food additives, I don't think the theory can be totally dismissed. Even the most critical of scientific groups has agreed that there may be a possibility that food colors affect some children. [23] However, I wholeheartedly agree with that same scientific group (American Council on Science and Health) that there are negative aspects of blaming a child's behavior on the food he or she eats. This can have long range complications. For example, in at least one case, a district judge has exonerated teenage juveniles of criminal charges, because he believed the junk food they ate was responsible for their behavior!

Since a food additive free diet causes no physical harm, there is certainly nothing wrong with parents giving it a try. Indeed, because food additives are highly associated with junk type foods, there may be some nutritional benefits. In the opinion of the author, it is in that light that the additive free diet should be presented to the child. Rather than emphasizing any effect it may have on his or her behavior, it should be emphasized that it is better for overall health. By avoiding foods containing additives, the child will also avoid a great many foods which contain what are known as "empty calories".

Any discussion of junk foods or "empty calories", of course, brings us to the subject of sugar. Certainly it is true that sugar has no pharmacological properties, and certainly it is true that sugar is only a source of carbohydrate. However, in the opinion of the author, it is relevant to point out that sugar is a highly concentrated source of carbohydrate . . . and that it is digested faster than any other food. Table sugar (sucrose) can increase the blood glucose level more rapidly than any other foodstuff. Recently it was reported in the American Journal of Clinical Nutrition that sugar may actually increase the metabolic rate (Figure 11-1). [26]

In animals, where behavior is readily detectable, it is well known that the energy content of feed can affect behavior. The best example of this is in horses. A goodly number of saddle horses are relatively calm and manageable when the only feed they receive consists of hay or pasture grass; that is, low energy

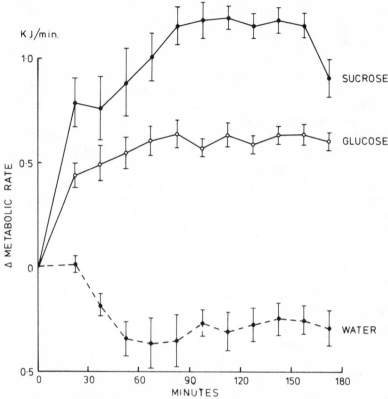

Figure 11-1. Metabolic rate as affected by sugar (sucrose) or starch (glucose). Sugar may be nothing but a carbohydrate, but it is digested faster than any other food. This data indicates it may increase the metabolic rate. (Reproduced with permission, Dr. N.N. Sharief, and Am. Journal of Clinical Nutrition.)

feeds. However, when fed grain (a high energy feed) they often become unruly and difficult to handle. While undocumented scientifically, the effect has literally been known for centuries, and is the source of the expression, "feeling his oats".

The use of sugar in prepared foods has increased rapidly over approximately the last 40 years. Occurring in approximately the same time frame, has been the reported increase in hyperactive children. Certainly this may be circumstantial, but in the author's opinion, it is relevant . . . especially when one considers that the amount of physical activity in children has declined over this same time period.

The situation is this; we have more and more children eating higher quantities of extremely high energy, rapidly assimilated foods . . . with declining constructive energy expenditures.

Modern children no longer have chores to do around the house or farm (if they do, it is with a power mower, rather than a push mower, etc.). Instead of playing baseball or football after school, the entertainment is often the 3:30/4:00 television cartoon show. Due to urban crime and traffic dangers, most children don't even walk or ride their bicycles to school anymore . . . they are chauffered, to and from.

This situation would be analogous to people who take a big dog, overfeed him, and then attempt to keep him penned up in a small backyard. The dog is going to dig holes, bark and howl, run and jump on people (playful or otherwise), and generally make a nuisance of himself.

Children have an innate desire to be active. (It is not until adolescence that they become accustomed to inactivity.) This is not to say that there are some children who may indeed have a psychological dysfunction that results in what is known as hyperkinesis. Again, looking at animals, we know this sort of thing exists. It is not uncommon to find individual horses who will literally run themselves to death. If not reined in, these horses, on their own volition, will run until they collapse. Certain individual dogs of the sporting breeds will also run until exhaustion drops them.

But for every animal that is difficult to control for purely psychological reasons, there are many more that simply suffer from a lack of exercise. The best example being the hobby horse that is kept penned up and ridden only once or twice a week. A horse that is unruly on Saturday afternoons, is often a different animal when taken to a working ranch. When ridden and worked every day, difficult horses typically become much more manageable.

In the author's opinion, this same analogy can be applied to children. If given some sort of physical exercise or work to do each day, or otherwise encouraged to participate in sports, much of their natural craving for activity will be vented. Likewise, it would seem prudent for parents to discourage the use of junk foods. At the present time there is no hard evidence that sugar or food additives are indeed involved in hyperactivity. But even if they are not, the child would benefit nutritionally.

Certainly these types of suggestions are not going to be totally effective for every rambunctious child. We know that some children do suffer from a dysfunction and need professional help. However, as a parent, I would damn sure do everything possible to allow my child to burn up his energy naturally, before turning to treatment with behavior altering drugs.

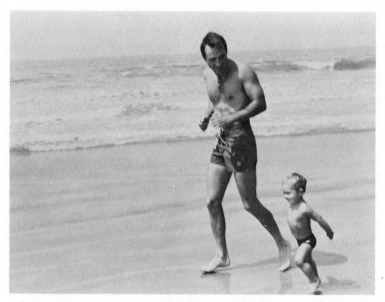

Figure 11-2. As a parent, I would do everything possible to allow my child to vent his energy, before submitting him to the use of behavior altering drugs.

Chapter 12   DIET AND DIABETES

Diet is believed to play a role in the onset of the adult form of diabetes.* (There are two commonly recognized forms of diabetes; juvenile onset, and adult onset.)

Juvenile onset diabetes is often called the insulin dependent type, since daily injections of insulin are usually required. The causes of juvenile diabetes are unknown. Genetics are believed to be involved, but do not totally explain incidences of the disease. This is because when identical twins are involved, only 50% of the time are both twins affected.[27]

It would seem then, that some type of environmental factor or factors are at least partially involved. One theory holds that certain viral infections may cause damage to the insulin producing cells of the pancreas. This theory is based on the fact that higher rates of juvenile diabetes have followed viral epidemics, and that individual juvenile diabetics have often been noted to have had certain serious viral diseases such as infectious mononucleosis.[28]

Diet is not believed to be a major factor in juvenile onset. It has been observed that affected children are often thin, but no common dietary factor has been identified.

Just the opposite is true for adult onset diabetes. While no single dietary nutrient has been identified, it is well known that obesity is a predisposing factor. In the U.S. there are an estimated 10 million diabetics, and of those diabetics, 9 million are believed to have been obesity induced.[29]

The exact reason obesity induces diabetes is not known, but there are a number of factors that could be involved. Diabetes, of course, is the inability to regulate blood glucose, commonly known as blood sugar. Insulin, the compound chiefly responsible for regulating blood glucose is secreted from the pancreas whenever the blood glucose level becomes too high. Insulin removes the glucose for uptake into the liver and other body cells.

Whenever a large amount of glucose rapidly appears in the blood, a rather high level of insulin is secreted (in normal people). Common table sugar is digested very quickly and is well known to produce unusually large insulin responses (as compared to other carbohydrates). For this reason, there have been attempts to associate sugar intake with diabetes, but to date, there has been no convincing evidence. Most of the evidence simply indicates sugar as a secondary factor related to obesity.

*Diabetes mellitus

Studies with primitive peoples indicate sugar as a disposing factor, but the evidence is purely circumstantial. That is, in their natural environment, diabetes is very rare among aboriginal peoples. When these groups, such as the Yemenite immigrants to Israel, African tribes,[29] and Eskimos,[30] etc. move into modern cities, diabetes becomes common. Because the traditional diets of these peoples contain very little sugar, but "civilized" diets are very high in sugar, a substantial correlation between sugar and diabetes can be drawn. However, as Dr. John Yudkin of the Univ. of London has pointed out, sucrose (table sugar), has only been around for about 200 years, but diabetes has been described in medical literature for over 3,000 years.[29] Indeed, it was the ancient Greeks that gave it its name, diabetes mellitus (Greek for sweet urine).

It would seem then, that sugar would tend to induce diabetes primarily through its substantial role in obesity. Primitive peoples are usually very lean in their natural environment, but experience has shown that they tend to be afflicted with obesity when the comforts and diet of modern civilization become available to them.

Still, (in the opinion of the author) sugar should not be ruled out entirely. Anything that can substantially affect insulin flow should remain suspect. Diabetes has been known for centuries, but the prevalence is increasing rapidly. Since 1967, the number of diabetics in the U.S. has doubled.[28]

However, obesity has also increased rapidly, and obesity itself can alter insulin flow. Obese people typically have higher circulating levels of insulin, and their body cells are usually not as responsive to insulin as leaner people. In addition, obese people tend to have higher levels of blood triglycerides. This could conceivably have an effect, since another major function of insulin is to remove fat (triglycerides) from the blood and deposit it into the tissues.

PHYSIOLOGICAL PROBLEMS FACED BY DIABETICS

The most well known danger faced by diabetics is hyperglycemia (excess glucose in the blood), which if unchecked, can lead to coma and death. Other problems faced by diabetics include greatly increased risk of atherosclerosis, reduced immunity to infectious diseases, and poor protein utilization.

Hyperglycemia is a constant source of danger to diabetics, but if the individual is faithful to his diet, careful about insulin injections (when required), and otherwise leads a prudent life, "diabetic shock" (hyperglycemia) need never occur. More unpredictable is the threat of coronary heart disease, precipitated by atherosclerosis.

As discussed on p. 104, diabetics are approximately five times more likely to suffer a coronary heart attack than non-diabetics. Most significantly, young women who are normally "protected" from atherosclerosis until menopause, are not protected when diabetic. The exact reasons diabetics are more susceptible are not known.

Diabetics often have elevated blood triglycerides which is what would be expected with low insulin (since insulin affects the removal of triglycerides from the blood into the fat tissues). Elevated triglycerides are also a positive risk factor in atherosclerosis. However, not all diabetics who suffer atherosclerosis have elevated triglycerides (or cholesterol).[31]

Poor protein utilization is the other problem faced by diabetics. Insulin plays a substantial role in protein formation, and when absent, a larger percentage of dietary protein is broken down for use as energy. In children, this can result in reduced growth. In both children and adults, it is believed that it results in reduced immunity to infectious diseases.[32] Reduced immunity is probably due to impaired formation of antibodies (see p. 71 & 72) and other anti-infection agents.

DIETS FOR DIABETICS

Because diabetes can vary with the individual, a general diet recommendation cannot be made. Only the attending physician should give individual diabetics dietary advice. In addition, at the present time there is a bit of controversy concerning what the relative levels of carbohydrate and fat in the diet should be.

There are two primary considerations that greatly conflict with one another. The first consideration is that carbohydrate should be minimized to reduce large glucose loads in the blood (necessitating insulin). However, if carbohydrate levels are reduced, then fat levels are usually increased. Because diabetics tend to have abnormally high blood lipid levels, and are predisposed to atherosclerosis, great care needs to be exercised when increasing the fat level in the diet.

In considering the question of fat in the diet, it should be pointed out that many diabetics are carbohydrate sensitive. That is, carbohydrates tend to increase blood triglyceride levels faster than dietary fats. For this reason, only a physician can prescribe a diet for an individual diabetic. The physician must assess the patient's sensitivity to carbohydrate, and from that information, arrive at a proper carbohydrate/fat ratio.

Other dietary advice will include discussion of the use of rapidly digested carbohydrates such as sugar. In most circumstances, the diabetic should avoid sugar and other forms of rapidly absorbed carbohydrate. Instead, the diabetic should rely on more slowly digested carbohydrates, such as potatoes, brown rice, whole wheat flour, etc. In certain instances, however, when the patient's blood glucose is very low, he or she may need to consume some sort of sugar. The physician's role is to teach the patient to recognize when this situation occurs, and to take appropriate action.

In most instances the physician will want the patient to achieve and maintain a lean bodyweight. Obviously, in the case of adult obesity induced diabetes, this will require a reducing type diet. However, due to problems associated with the inability to regulate blood glucose, the patient should be very careful about dieting, and should not make any significant dietary changes unless directed by the physician.

Whatever the type of diet prescribed by the physician, in nearly all instances the patient will be instructed to eat several small meals a day, rather than just 3 large ones. This is to spread glucose release into the blood over a longer period of time. Large meals tend to jump the blood glucose levels rather high, which of course, necessitates the need for insulin. By eating smaller meals, and snacks in between, the need for insulin is moderated.

In summary, it should be re-emphasized that large metabolic differences occur between diabetics, and that only the attending physician familiar with the patient, is in a position to make specific recommendations.

DIET IN THE PREVENTION OF DIABETES

Since diabetes is known to have strong genetic implications, diet alone cannot be totally protective. However, it is believed that in many instances genetics simply predisposes the individual to diabetes; that is, makes the individual more susceptible to environmental influences. This is particularly true for adult, obesity onset diabetes. It follows then, that prudent dietary practices could probably reduce the number of diabetics, but not eliminate diabetes entirely.

Quite obviously, the avoidance of overeating would do much to eliminate the onset of obesity induced adult diabetes. There is also some indication that a moderate exercise program (in people who would otherwise be sedentary) would also tend to be protective of diabetes. Exercise tends to reduce the amount of circulating insulin, and also apparently enables muscle cells to absorb at least some glucose without the aid of insulin.

While this idea is controversial, it is the author's opinion that the avoidence of sugar would be protective. As mentioned previously, sugar precipitates large and sudden releases of insulin, although it has never been conclusively proven that these extraordinary mobilizations of insulin are detrimental. Even if they are not detrimental, however, a reduction of sugar intake would reduce inclination to obesity - which, of course, would be protective in itself.

In relation to juvenile onset diabetes, probably the only thing that could be recommended would be general good health and hygiene practices. If juvenile diabetes is indeed caused by viral infections, then a program of good basic nutrition, moderate exercise, and plenty of rest would be advised. It is important to remember that antibiotics are not effective against viruses (see p. 70). The only way a child (or any living creature) can combat a viral infection is through the body's own natural immunity system. Therefore to prevent or reduce the impact of serious viral infections, parents should see to it that their children eat balanced meals, and do not get physically "run down".

Chapter 13 HYPERTENSION (HIGH BLOOD PRESSURE)

As the reader is well aware, high blood pressure is a very serious and common ailment. Persons with medically defined hypertension are much more likely to suffer heart attacks and strokes than people with normal blood pressure values (see Figure 13-1).

Hypertension is usually classified as being either of a primary or a secondary type. The secondary type refers to situations in which there is a known specific cause. These causes may be physical or hormonal. The most common physical causes usually entail some sort of arterial constriction at the kidney. There are also a number of hormonal imbalances which can cause arterial constriction. Again, the kidneys are often the site of these constrictions.

Primary hypertension. The primary type of hypertension is one in which there is no apparent cause. There is no single area within the circulatory system or identifiable hormone that is causing the blood pressure to be elevated.

The primary type of hypertension has been the subject of much concern, because it is believed that some of the underlying causes are preventable. One of the best known factors, obesity, is quite obviously preventable or reversable. The effects caused by psycological stress, anger, or frustration may or may not be preventable or reversable.

Most of the current discussion concerning primary hypertension has centered around excessive salt consumption. As early as 1904, salt was implicated as a predisposing factor.[33] However, concern over salt has intensified recently, because of the widespread use of salt in virtually all prepared foods. Unless all meals are prepared at home (from unprocessed food), it is practically impossible to avoid eating an excessive amount of salt.

The National Research Council has determined that 3 grams of salt [33] (½ teaspoon) would more than meet the needs of most adults. (Actual requirements have been calculated to be as low as .5 gram.[5]) Yet actual consumption in the U.S. has been found to vary from 6 to 17 grams (1 to 3 teaspoons). [34] In northern Japan, salt consumption is on the order of 20-25 grams/day. [33]

Overconsumption of salt is nothing new. Throughout history man has used salt both as a preservative and a condiment. The Romans even paid their soldiers salt as part of their wages, which became the source of the word "salary".

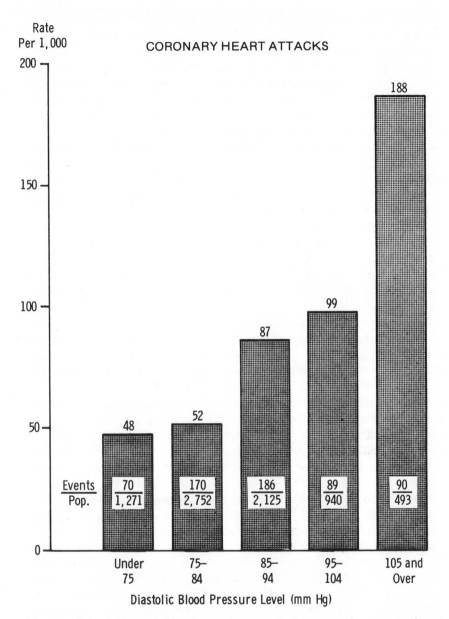

Figure 13-1. Effect of blood pressure on incidences of coronary heart attacks. Source: DHEW Pub. No. 72-219.

Not all people develop high blood pressure as a result of excess salt consumption. In the U.S. it is estimated that only 20% of the population actually suffer from hypertension.[5] Because of this, it is believed that there is a genetic factor involved. That is, certain people are more susceptible to salt excesses than others. This theory has been demonstrated with laboratory animals. Strains of salt-hypertension susceptible and resistant rats have been developed by feeding high levels of salt. It should be pointed out, however, that at extremely high levels of salt intake, approximately 80% of all rats develop hypertension.

The exact mechanism by which salt increases blood pressure is not accurately known. It is generally accepted that salt increases what is known as extracellular pressure which would tend to constrict the blood vessels. However, there may be more to it than that.

There has been at least one research report that has indicated that arteries from people afflicted with hypertension may actually have a higher salt (sodium) content than arteries from normal people. In regard to this, there has been speculation that this may cause a thickening of the arterial wall, and thereby create a constriction.[35]

This theory, however, has not been proven. Still, in the opinion of the author, it should be cause for some thought, and possible concern. If some sort of mechanism like this is involved, it means that reduced salt intake will not totally reverse the situation. Indeed, in many cases of primary hypertension, drug treatment is required in addition to a low salt (sodium) diet, and even drugs are not always effective at lowering blood pressure to normal levels. Also, there are reports that in primitive peoples who have a very low salt intake, blood pressure does not increase with age. (In developed countries, blood pressure increases gradually with age.)

The Food and Nutrition Board of the National Academy of Sciences has reported that hypertension is absent in primitive peoples that typically consume very little salt. Studies report that the populations of the Soloman Islands, the Coco Islands of Polynesia, and certain Indian tribes of the Amazon Basin consume only about 2 grams of salt per day, and essentially have no hypertension.[33] This, plus the fact that there is no known benefit to eating excess salt, has led the National Research Council to recommend that the public as a whole reduce their consumption of salt.

Three grams per day has been set as the goal. According to the National Research Council, to achieve this goal the use of salt in cooking and at the table would have to be eliminated. If prepared foods are used, however, it may be impossible to limit intake to 3 grams. (Commercially prepared foods not only contain extra salt, but often contain sodium based additives as well; e.g. monosodium glutamate, sodium benzoate, sodium propionate, etc.) Table 13-1 is a comparison of the salt content of a number of commercially prepared foods and the unprocessed product they are made from.

Cutting down on salt. Unless you already have high blood pressure, there is no need to go on a crash low sodium diet. Indeed, since sodium is intimately involved with body metabolism, it is probably best to cut down slowly. Start by not salting foods at the table. Then proceed to gradually cut down on prepared foods, cured meats, etc. that contain added salt.

Once you begin cutting down, unsalted foods will taste rather bland. However, after a while they will begin to taste more normal. Ultimately, you will become much more sensitive to the salt taste and commercially salted food will taste disagreeably salty.

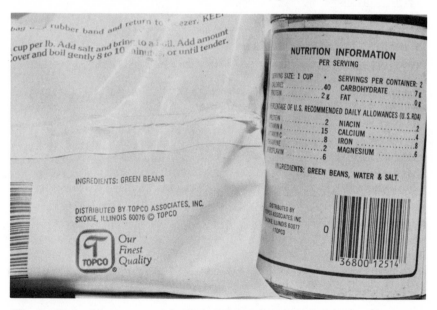

Figure 13-2. Most canned foods contain salt, whereas frozen foods typically do not.

Special needs. During periods of extensive sweating, it is generally recognized that salt requirements are increased. Extreme muscular exertion during the summer or otherwise in a hot environment, can result in sweat losses of up to 1½ quarts per hour. According to the National Research Council, whenever more than about

TABLE 13-1. SALT EQUIVALENT IN SELECTED PREPARED FOODS.*

	Serving Size	Salt Equivqlent**
Beef:		
Cooked, lean	3 ounces	138 milligrams
Corned	3 oz	2005
Bologna	3 oz	1650
Fish:		
Catfish	3 oz	125
Canned tuna	3 oz	758
Shrimp, raw	3 oz	343
Shrimp, canned	3 oz	4888
Pork:		
Fresh, cooked lean	3 oz	148
Ham	3 oz	2785
Sausage	3 oz	2520
Prepared Dishes		
Chili con carne w/beans, canned regular	1 cup	2985
canned low sodium	1 cup	250
Pizza, frozen	7 oz (½pie)	2033
Ravioli, canned	7.5 oz	2663
Spagetti sauce, canned	4 oz	2140
Stew, canned	8 oz	2450
Chicken dinner (frozen TV dinner)	1 dinner	2883
Grain Products		
White bread, regular	1 slice	285
low sodium	1 slice	17.5
Breakfast cereals :		
Oatmeal, regular	3/4 cup	450
low sodium	3/4 cup	2.5
Cornflakes, regular	1 cup	640
low sodium	1 cup	20
Vegetables		
Asparagus, fresh or frozen	4 spears	10
canned	4 spears	745
Cabbage, fresh	1 cup	20
sauerkraut, canned	1 cup	3885
Peas, fresh	1 cup	5
canned	1 cup	1232

*USDA Salt in your food
**Extrapolated from sodium content (for sodium content only, multiply salt equivalent times .4).

3 quarts of water are required to replace sweat losses, extra salt is justified. The recommended amount varies from 2 to 7 grams per quart, depending upon the individual. People who are not accustomed to heavy sweating would tend to lose more sodium, and therefore would need the higher level of salt. Conversely, steel workers, coal miners, etc., who are otherwise accustomed to high temperatures and/or heavy sweating would probably tend to lose less sodium and therefore require less salt.

Chapter 14   NUTRITIONAL ASPECTS OF HEART DISEASE

THE CHOLESTEROL CONTROVERSY

At the present time there is an enormous disparity of opinion concerning the effect of cholesterol and saturated fats in the diet. The fundamental basis for the controversy is the fact that there is relatively little known concerning the metabolism of cholesterol and fats in humans. The issue at controversy, of course, is the effect dietary fats and cholesterol have upon atherosclerosis and subsequent heart disease.

Atherosclerosis. Atherosclerosis is a condition whereby compounds containing cholesterol and other fatty constituents are deposited in the arteries. Occurring over a substantial period of time, the deposits can eventually cause a constriction within the artery. Ultimately they can cause the heart to work harder (to pump blood through the constriction). In addition, for some yet unknown reason, blood clots often form at the site of constriction. When this happens, of course, it can be a life threatening situation.

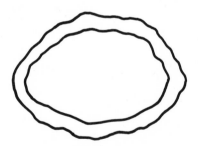 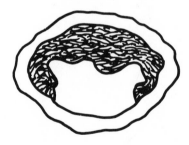

14-1a   14-1b

Figure 14-1a and 14-1b. Normal artery (1a), and artery blocked by atherosclerosis(1b). Fibrous plaques consisting of fats and cholesterol become deposited in the arterial wall during atherosclerosis. These blockages can become an impediment to blood flow. For some unknown reason it is also believed they tend to cause blood clots at the point of constriction, which can quite obviously be a life threatening situation.

Atherosclerosis is nothing new. As pointed out by the American Council on Science and Health, in his original investigations into human anatomy, Leonardo de Vinci made the observation that man is "only as old as his arteries"[36]. Figures 14-2 and 14-3 are photographs of arteries dissected from Egyptian mummies which show evidence of blockage.

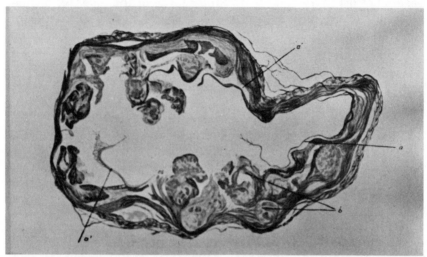

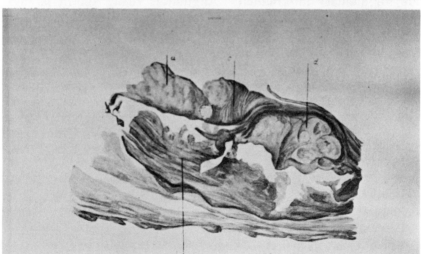

Figure 14-2. Sections of arteries taken from Egyptian mummies showing evidence of blockage. (Photo courtesy of Dr. Elizabeth Whelan, American Council on Science and Health. Original source, M.A. Ruffer. Studies in the Paleopathology of Egypt. Univ. of Chicago Press. 1921.)

But while the identification of atherosclerosis as a disease entity is nothing new, its rate of identification and diagnosis is. That is, coronary heart disease as caused by atherosclerosis has become the leading cause of death in the U.S. and other developed countries.

Because of its obvious importance, there has been an intense research effort to try and identify the causes of the disease. While advances have been made, in actuality there is very little known.

By observation it is known that fatty streaks within the arteries may appear as early as infancy. The National Health Institute's Task Force on Arteriosclerosis has reported that by the age of 10, fatty streaks are present in the aorta of every child regardless of race, sex, or environment.[31] Autopsies performed on combat soldiers killed in Korea and Viet Nam have shown that lesions can appear in young adulthood and are relatively common. [37,38] It is generally (but not universally) believed that the fibrous plaques associated with atherosclerosis are an advancement of the fatty streaks universally seen in children.[31]

Knowing that fatty streaks are present in all populations, the unanswered question remains, "Why do lesions of life endangering proportions develop in some people, and in others regress or remain harmless". To date, research has only been able to provide fragmentary information. All that is really known is that there are a number of risk factors that will tend to increase the likelihood of atherosclerosis in a given individual.

TABLE 14-1. RISK FACTORS.[31]

1. Age
2. Male sex (women are protected until after menapause).
3. Elevated blood lipid values (cholesterol and triglycerides)
4. Hypertension (high blood pressure)
5. Cigarette smoking
6. Impaired glucose tolerance (diabetes)
7. Obesity
8. Physical inactivity
9. Personality and behavior
10. Family history (genetics)
11. Gout
12. Hardness of drinking water (soft water being positive: hardwater, negative)

Of these risk factors, elevated blood cholesterol has by far received the greatest attention. This is no doubt due to the fact that blood lipid values can be modified though the use of restrictive diets and drugs.

The compound. Cholesterol is a compound synthesized within the body that is used as a building block for numerous physiological compounds. The most notable of which being the sex hormones. Cholesterol is the basis for a large number of sterols and hormones used in the body which we could not function without.

Because cholesterol is vital to animal life, then obviously it is contained in the animal products that we use for food. Table 14-2 is a listing of the levels of cholesterol contained in various foods (in decreasing order).

Food	Cholesterol content per 100 g edible portion
Egg yolk	1,500 mg
Egg, whole	550
Liver	300
Butter	250
Oysters	200
Lobster	200
Shrimp & crabmeat	125
Cheese (cheddar)	100
Beef	70
Fish	70
Lamb	70
Pork	70
Chicken	60
Cottage cheese (creamed)	15
Milk, (fluid, whole)	11
Milk, (fluid, skim)	3

TABLE 14-2. CHOLESTEROL CONTENT OF COMMON FOODS (in descending order). Source: USDA Nutritive Value of Foods. Book No. 8.

Although current research has not been able to provide detailed answers to the many questions concerning dietary cholesterol, it has been successful in bringing us to the realization that cholesterol metabolism is an extremely complex situation.

Early research. Early research was primarily conducted with laboratory animals and patients who had a history of heart disease. In 1913 it was shown that when rabbits were fed a high cholesterol diet, they would develop fatty lesions within the arteries. Later work showed that chickens would develop similar lesions. Early in the 1940's there were studies to show that groups of heart patients suffering coronary heart disease tended to have elevated blood cholesterol, although many had completely normal values.[31] When patients with elevated blood cholesterol values were put on low fat, low cholesterol diets, in a majority of cases, blood cholesterol levels decreased. This information was the basis for the physicians and scientists who began recommending that the public as a whole cut down on fats and cholesterol.

Later research with laboratory animals. Later research showed that there were great differences between species, in regard to response to high cholesterol diets. In rabbits, chickens, and rhesus monkeys, fatty streaks within the arteries could be demonstrated by feeding high cholesterol diets. In rats and dogs there was no response. It was found that in order for lesions to appear in rats and dogs, thyroid activity had to be depressed. Diet alone had no effect.

Of the animals susceptible to the formation of fatty lesions, it was found that the lesions would regress, when the animals were returned to their normal diet. However, in reviewing the scientific literature on animal research, the National Health Institute's Task Force on Arteriosclerosis reported that only rarely did the lesions produced in animals develop into the fibrous plaques associated with heart disease in man.[31]

Cholesterol metabolism in man. Very little is actually known about the metabolism of cholesterol in man. As mentioned earlier, cholesterol is a necessity for normal body function, and it is known that the body can synthesize cholesterol, even if the diet contains no cholesterol or fats whatsoever. Most cholesterol synthesis occurs in the liver, although nearly all body cells are also capable of synthesizing the compound.

If cholesterol is added to the diet, the synthesis of cholesterol within the body is suppressed (in normal individuals). Normally it takes a period of time for the suppression of cholesterol synthesis to occur. That is, when people are on a low cholesterol diet and then suddenly begin eating high levels of cholesterol, it takes about 2 to 3 weeks before their bodies become adjusted by lowering cholesterol synthesis. Because it takes a period of time for the body to reduce cholesterol synthesis, blood cholesterol levels will be abnormally high during the interim period. [39]

Suppression of cholesterol synthesis during intake of high levels of cholesterol is not complete. Persons consuming low cholesterol diets will have a modestly lower blood cholesterol value, than if they were on a higher level of cholesterol intake. [32]

Recent research. The most recent research has shown that the form in which cholesterol is transported in the blood has a great deal to do with the tendency toward atherosclerosis. High levels of one type have been statistically proven to be a positive risk factor, while high levels of another type actually appear to be protective.

Cholesterol is transported through the blood by specialized carrier proteins called lipoproteins. (Lipo, of course, means fat; hence the term lipo/protein.) These proteins are classified according to their density. The most important ones (in respect to atherosclerosis) are Low-Density Lipoproteins and High Density Lipoproteins.

Increased levels of Low-Density Lipoproteins have been shown to be a positive risk factor for atherosclerosis. Conversely, relatively high levels of High-Density Lipoproteins have been shown to be protective of cardiovascular problems. [40,41,31,32]

High blood cholesterol. For undetermined reasons, some people have abnormally high blood cholesterol levels. Known as hyper-cholesterolemia, these people are much more prone to atherosclerosis than people with normal values. The dangerously high level is generally accepted to be about 250 milligrams per liter of blood. As can be seen from Figure 14-3, people with blood cholesterol values of over 250 mg. have a much higher risk of heart attack.

As mentioned, it is not understood why certain individuals are predisposed to abnormally high levels . At least one medical researcher has mentioned that it may be a hormonal disturbance. His basis for this thought is the fact that women are apparently "protected" until the onset of menapause. [41] Another theory might be thyroid dysfunction. That is, it has been demonstrated that thyroid activity must be depressed to create the condition

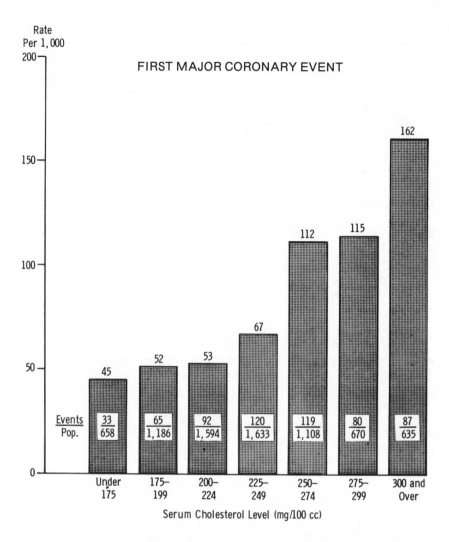

Figure 14-3. Blood cholesterol level in men as related to the first major coronary event (heart attack). Source: DHEW Pub. No. 72-219.

in certain laboratory animals, then possibly a thyroid irregularity might be a factor in man.

Although the exact physiological cause is not known, it is generally agreed that genetics plays a substantial role. A researcher with the National Heart, Lung, and Blood Institute has pointed out that for one type of inherited hypercholesterolemia, subjects frequently develop coronary problems as early as age 15.[42] Blood cholesterol problems have been detected in infants as early as 5 days after birth. In one particular instance, a breastfed youngster was shown to have a blood cholesterol level that would be considered abnormally high in a 70 year old man [43] (blood cholesterol levels increase with age).

Looking at coronary disease itself, persons with a family history of the problem have a much greater chance of developing coronary problems than the public at large. In a study conducted in London, the families of 200 coronary patients were studied. It was found that the men under age 55 and the women under age 65 had a seven fold increase in the risk of death from a coronary heart attack. [31]

In respect to hypercholesterolemia, the same genetic aspects seen in man, have been demonstrated with animals. In a comprehensive study with squirrel monkeys, certain lines showed sharply increased blood cholesterol differences on high fat diets, while others showed only modest increases. The researchers determined that the heritability for blood cholesterol was approximately 90%. [31]

Dietary recommendations for hypercholesterolemia. It is generally recommended that people with high blood cholesterol levels should consume low cholesterol diets. In addition, dietary fats are usually restricted, particularly saturated or animal fats. Saturated fats tend to enhance the absorption of cholesterol. Unsaturated or vegetable fats do not tend to increase the absorption of cholesterol. However, vegetable fats that have been hydrogenated* do enhance the absorption of cholesterol. [44]

In many cases dietary restriction of fats and cholesterol is not effective in lowering blood cholesterol to normal levels. Drugs are required in addition to diet therapy. [45,31,42] That is, in many people afflicted with hypercholesterolemia, their bodies synthesize excess cholesterol, and reducing dietary cholesterol is not effective. Drugs that suppress synthesis are required.

Dietary recommendation for normal people. At the present time, the subject of dietary recommendations for normal people is an enormously controversial issue. There are some scientific/medical groups that believe that it would be wise for the public in general

---

*Hydrogenation is the hardening process used in making margarine and shortening. By adding hydrogen, vegetable oils can be made hard so they can be put in a stick (have the consistency of butter or lard).

to consume low cholesterol diets; substituting vegetable oils for animal fats. Other scientific groups have pointed out that there is no evidence that restictive diets would benefit people with normal blood cholesterol values.

Probably the most valid criticism is that such a move would yield a false sense of security to people at risk for atherosclerosis. The public as a whole would get the idea that dietary cholesterol is synonymous with atherosclerosis, when in fact dietary restrictions are often not effective in lowering hypercholesterol levels to more normal levels. That is, people afflicted with hypercholesterolemia might not seek out proper medical help for drug treatment, in addition to the dietary treatment they need. (Further discussion is continued on p. 108.)

OTHER DIETARY FACTORS

Sugar. There are elements within the scientific community that have suggested sugar as a possible contributing factor to heart disease. Dr. John Yudkin, professor emeritus of Queen Elizabeth College in London, has been the primary advocate.

As Dr. Yudkin has pointed out, primitive peoples are not afflicted with the so-called diseases of affluent society. Atherosclerosis, diabetes, hypertension and several other metabolic disturbances occur only rarely in most primitive cultures. These types of physiological problems begin to occur only when primitive peoples come into contact with "civilization" and the soda pop, candy and confectionary foods that are so readily available.

On the average, affluent societies eat substantially more animal protein and fats than less developed cultures. In many cases it has therefore been assumed that animal products have been responsible for atherosclerosis. However, Dr. Yudkin points out that not all primitive societies eat reduced amounts of animal products. On the contrary, there are primitive societies whose dietary intake is made up almost entirely of animal proteins and fats. The Masai and Samburu tribesmen of East Africa maintain extensive herds of cattle and eat a diet based on milk, blood, and meat. There are a number of nomadic tribes in the Middle East that eat substantial amounts of goat milk, meat, and mutton. There are the Laplanders of Finland, Sweden, and Siberia whose diet is based on the reindeer herds they have maintained for centuries. Then, of course, there are the Eskimos whose diet consists almost entirely of seal and whale meat, blubber, and fish.

Although the evidence is circumstantial, it does seem significant that these peoples do not suffer atherosclerosis and diabetes,

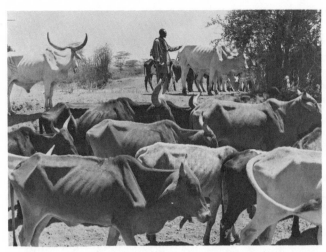

(Figure 14-4 by F. Botts, courtesy of Winter Photographic Safaris, P.O. Box 24871, Nairobi Kenya. Figure 14-5 courtesy of the government of Finland.)

Figure 14-4 & 14-5. Coronary heart disease is rare among primitive peoples, yet some primitive peoples consume diets high in animal fat and cholesterol. Pictured above is a Masai tribesman of East Africa tending the cattle they have mainained for centuries. Cattle blood and milk is the mainstay of the diet, which is higher in choesterol than the diet of any other people in the world. Pictured below are the Laplanders of Finland working reindeer that have been the mainstay of their diet since recorded history.

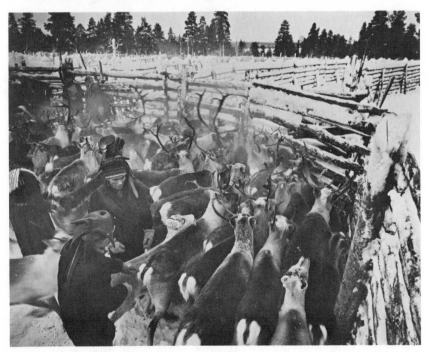

etc., until they come into contact with modern civilization. When this happens, their consumption of animal protein often actually decreases, whereas their intake of sugar increases enormously.

What causes some scientists to dispute the sugar/atherosclerosis theory is that increased sugar consumption does not ordinarily increase the blood cholesterol level. However, it is well known that highly refined carbohydrates will increase the blood triglyceride level.[31] Triglycerides are a form of fat, which are also known to be a positive risk factor for coronary disease. Of the carbohydrates, sugar creates the greatest triglyceride increase.

Sugar (sucrose) also modifies insulin secretion. This may be of importance, since it is well documented that diabetics are much more likely to suffer coronary heart attacks that non-diabetics. In diabetic men, age 15 to 44, the death rate for coronary heart disease is 4.6 times higher than for non-diabetic men, and in diabetic women the rate is 6.4 times higher. It is interesting to note that pre-menapausal diabetic women are not "protected" from atherosclerosis like non-diabetic women. In one large study, vascular disease was responsible for 75% of the deaths in the diabetic study group.[31]

Dr. Otto Schaefer, a Canadian medical researcher studying the Eskimos of the Northwest Territories, reported a number of disorders common only to the Eskimos that have come into contact with civilization and sugary foods. Like other reports and researchers of primitive peoples, he reported remarkable increases in the incidences of diabetes, gall bladder disease, dental caries (cavities), and atherosclerosis.[30,46] Dr. Schaefer used a rather novel, and interesting approach. He developed a graph relating tooth decay to the incidence of arterial calcification. As the amount of tooth decay increased, the incidences of atherosclerosis increased at a similar rate (see Figure 14-6a & b).

As Dr. Schaefer explained, tooth decay most obviously does not cause atherosclerosis. However, it does demonstrate the presence of a third factor . . . sugar. In their native environment, Eskimos never brush their teeth. Since they eat essentially no sugar, dental hygiene isn't necessary. Tooth brushing not being a customary practice, the introduction of civilized foods has resulted in substantial tooth decay. It (tooth decay) is therefore a reasonably good indication of sugar intake.

In studying the metabolic responses of Eskimos to sugar, Dr. Schaefer points out that the relationships may not be directly applicable to other peoples, since the Eskimo's introduction to sugar has been extraordinarily sudden. As Dr. Schaefer explains, the traditional diet contained only inconsequential amounts of

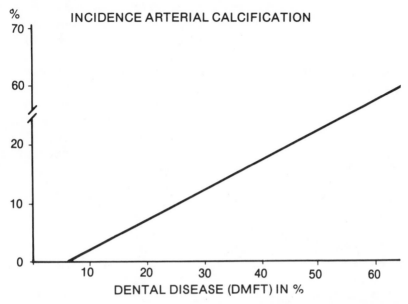

INCIDENCE ARTERIAL CALCIFICATION

DENTAL DISEASE (DMFT) IN %

Figures 14-6a & b. Dr. Otto Schaefer, a Canadian medical researcher found an indirect relationship between sugar and atherosclerosis in Eskimos. In their native environment, Eskimos consume essentially no sugar, and therefore dental hygiene is not necessary, and is not practiced. When the Eskimos become a part of "civilization", they begin consuming large amounts of sugar, and in the absence of dental hygiene, tooth decay is a direct indicator of sugar intake. Dr. Schaefer found that tooth decay was a relatively good indicator of arteriosclerosis. Whenever tooth decay was high, X-ray examination of the arteries also revealed a high incidence of arteriosclerosis. Photo and graph courtesy of Dr. Otto Schaefer.

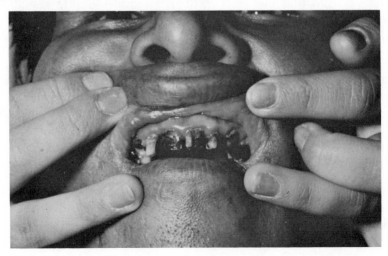

readily absorbable carbohydrate. The only sugar they got was what was contained in the occasional berries they were able to find. The only other glucose like carbohydrates available to the Eskimo were the glycoproteins contained in whale skin ("muk tuk"), and glycogen contained in the liver. The vegetable matter in the diet was restricted to "roots, leaf greens, and seaweed". By far, the majority of the energy (calories) in the diet came from protein.

Dr. Schaefer is, of course, correct in pointing out how rapid the introduction to sugar has been. He explains that the Eskimo could not have had the opportunity for a genetic adaptation to sugar in the diet, and the abnormal insulin responses it causes.

In the author's opinion, however, it should be pointed out that while the Eskimo's introduction to sugar has indeed been extraordinarily sudden . . . in terms of the known history of man's existence on this planet, the introduction of sugar to the human race in general has also been extremely sudden. That is, modern man dates back for at least 40,000 years.[47] Yet as Dr. Yudkin has pointed out, sugar did not become part of the diet until slave trade began between West Africa and the Carribean in the 1800's. Less than 200 years ago sugar consumption consisted of only 4 lbs. per year in the diet of European peoples. Today, the average consumption of sugar is 120 lbs. It is also important to realize that only 40 years ago, sugar consumption was only half of what it is today.[48]

Whether we talk about primitive peoples recently encompassed by civilization, or "civilized" man himself, there has been a precipitous increase in sugar consumption. In terms of man's existence on earth, sugar has only been available for a split second in time. The variable that makes it difficult to draw definite conclusions, is the vast difference in physical activity between primitive and affluent societies. Primitive peoples are much more active and exposed to more environmental physical stress than civilized peoples, and certainly this is protective of heart disease. We can look at the constituents of the diets of primitive peoples before and after merging into civilization, but we must also look at total caloric intake. Overeating and obesity typically occur among primitive peoples in "civilized" societies. This, coupled with physical inactivity, makes it very difficult to say whether the "primitive" diet was protective, or the "civilized" diet is causative.

Alcohol. Alcohol is known to increase both blood triglycerides and cholesterol. In addition, alcohol is known to adversely affect the physiology of the heart directly.[10,49]

The reason blood triglycerides and cholesterol are increased by alcohol is believed to be related to the damage alcohol does to the liver. A major function of the liver is to synthesize triglycerides and cholesterol. It is postulated that alcohol tends to inhibit the ability of the liver to metabolize (burn up) fats, while abnormally increasing the synthesis of fats. These fats are believed to be either deposited in the liver (contribute to fatty liver syndrome), or released to the blood, thereby creating abnormally high blood lipid values.

Diabetics are particularly susceptible to elevated blood lipids due to alcohol. Also, people who already have tendencies toward hypertriglycerides and cholesterol due to a carbohydrate insensitivity*, will be more radically affected by alcohol.[10]

The effect of alcohol upon atherosclerosis itself remains somewhat controversial. A confounding factor may be that in severe cases of alcoholism where liver damage is extensive, blood lipids are actually reduced. Whether this means that cirrhosis is protective of atherosclerosis is not clear, but it does seem that it would tend to make it difficult to obtain a simple statistical correlation. Given the fact that alcohol does increase blood lipids, and given the number of people who ingest alcohol daily (usually in the evening with the heaviest meal of the day), it would seem that alcohol could indeed be a factor in atherosclerosis.

Cigarette smoking. Whether smoking can be considered a dietary factor is certainly open to question. However, there can be no question but that smoking is indeed a factor contributing to heart disease.

Smoking contributes to virtually every aspect of coronary disease, but none of the mechanisms are clearly understood. One of the most puzzling aspects is that smoking apparently contributes to atherosclerosis itself. How it is able to do that is not known, but studies with laboratory animals have shown that exposure to carbon monoxide increases the severity of atherosclerosis.[50]

It is also thought that cigarette smoke tends to increase the likelihood of blood clotting.[51] When a blood clot forms in the area of a lesion (from atherosclerosis), the artery can become plugged, and a coronary heart attack is much more likely to occur.

Adding to the likelihood of a coronary, is the well known ability of cigarette smoking to elevate blood pressure. This, coupled with the fact that nicotine increases the heart rate, makes cigarette smoking a very substantial risk factor in heart disease.

*There are a number of people who develop abnormal blood triglycerides and cholesterol due to a high carbohydrate diet (particularly refined carbohydrates).

But not only do cigarette smokers have a much greater likelihood of suffering a heart attack in the first place . . . they also have a greatly reduced chance of surviving the attack once it occurs. Presumably this is due to the fact that smoking decreases the ability of the blood to carry and exchange oxygen.[31]

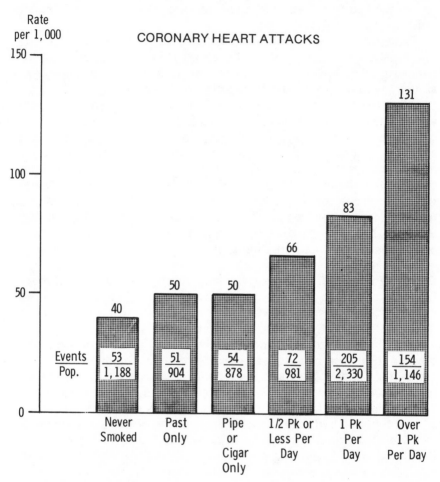

Figure 14-7. Cigarette smoking and age-adjusted rates of first major coronary event for white males (age 30-59). Source: DHEW Pub. No. 72-219.

CONCLUSIONS ON HEART DISEASE AND DIET

It is clear that there is a segment of the population afflicted with hypercholesterolemia (abnormally high blood cholesterol levels). People with cholesterol levels above 250 mg./100 ml. of blood are known to be at substantially greater risk for athero-sclerosis and heart disease. Elevated blood triglyceride levels also are a positive risk factor. People with blood triglyceride levels of over 200 mg./100 ml. blood are at increased risk, regardless of the blood cholesterol level. That is, blood triglyceride levels are a risk factor independent of blood cholesterol values.

Marginally high blood cholesterol and triglyceride levels are often due to simple obesity and overeating. Reducing intake and weight loss will often correct the situation. Weight loss not only reduces total blood cholesterol and triglycerides, but also increases the proportion of high-density lipoprotein cholesterol, which is known to be protective of heart disease.

It is almost unanimously agreed that persons with abnormally high blood cholesterol levels should consume low fat/cholesterol diets. Although it has never been conclusively proven that mod-ifying the diet of hypercholesterolemic patients is actually effective in reducing the onset or severity of coronary disease, it is almost universally agreed that it should be done. Blood cholesterol levels over 250 mg. are indeed abnormally high, and reducing them to normal values does appear to be a logical thing to do. There is essentially no argument or controversy concerning this matter.

The controversy begins when one considers diet recommend-ations for normal people. The American Heart Association is of the opinion that the public should be told to reduce consumption of animal fats and cholesterol and increase the consumption of unsaturated vegetable fats. This view has been apposed by a number of scientific groups.

There are several reasons for opposition to this type of blanket recommendation. Probably the most significant is that it leads the public as a whole to the conclusion that coronary disease has a simple cause and effect relationship. "High blood cholesterol is the cause of heart disease, and if you eat reduced amounts of animal fats, then you won't get heart disease". This, of course, is a gross oversimplification, and is potentially dangerous.

The most dangerous aspect of this conclusion is that it gives a false sense of security to those who are at risk of coronary disease due to hypercholesterolemia, and/or increased blood triglycerides. As discussed previously, for patients suffering from hypercholes-terolemia, diet therapy alone is often not enough. Hypercholesterol-emia is a metabolic disorder, and in many cases drugs are required, in addition to diet therapy. That is, restrictive diets alone, are often not effective in lowering blood cholesterol levels to normal values.

The fear, of course, is that a portion of the population will not avail themselves for medical examination (thinking that all they need do is eat lean meat, margarine instead of butter, avoid egg yolks, etc.). As a result, many people with hypercholesterolemia will fail to be identified and receive proper preventative treatment.

This type of thinking holds an even greater danger for people with elevated triglycerides. As discussed previously, carbohydrates are capable of increasing blood triglyceride values at a greater rate than fats (readily available carbohydrates, such as sugar, in particular). In addition, there are some people who are particularly sensitive to carbohydrates, but tolerate fats quite well. If these people were to reduce their consumption of fats and increase their consumption of carbohydrates, it could be to their detriment.

For this reason, the American Medical Association has adopted the position that acknowledges the existence of people with hyperlipemia (abnormally high blood cholesterol, and/or triglycerides). Rather than make a simple dietary recommendation, the AMA suggests that everyone consult a physician and have a blood profile analysis taken. In this way, if cholesterol or triglycerides are in excess, the cause may be identified and treated properly.[52]

As for dietary recommendations, the National Research Council (NRC) suggests that the public simply eat a balanced diet, being careful to maintain total caloric intake within actual energy needs. NRC warns against overeating of any type of foodstuff (fats, protein, or carbohydrate) as overeating and obesity in general can increase blood lipid values, and is itself a risk factor. At this time, the NRC feels it unwise to make specific nutrient recommendations, such as substituting unsaturated vegetable oils for saturated animal fats. The longterm consequences of such a move are simply not known, and the NRC points out that making dietary recommendations without adequate scientific information, could actually be detrimental instead of beneficial.[33]

Commenting along these lines, Dr. Yudkin of the Univ. of London, has pointed out that vegetable oils have been with us for less than 100 years. It was not until the Industrial Revolution, that the ability to extract oil from soybeans, cottonseeds, sunflower, etc. became possible. Indeed, it has only been about the last 50 years that they have been available in any quantity. Dr. Yudkin argues that animal fat has been part of the human diet for nearly two million years, and to make a sudden switch to vegetable fat could be unwise, since we really don't know what other effects it might have.[41]

The scientific information that is available, can be used to support both sides of the argument. It is known that some vegetable oils such as safflower and soybean, will reduce total blood cholesterol values. This is the basis for the National Heart Association's recommendations. However, it is also known that when vegetable oils are hydrogenated*, they actually increase the absorption of cholesterol. Again, the public at large would receive a false sense of security. Margarine and vegetable shortening manufacturers often advertise their products as cholesterol free, high in polyunsaturates, etc., but in actuality, because the oils contained in them have been hydrogenated, they are in reality capable of enhancing cholesterol absorption. Other oils, such as coconut oil (commonly used in imitation dairy products, infant formulas, etc.), are able to promote cholesterol absorption in their liquid (unhydrogentated) state.[53]

Scientific trials conducted by the National Heart Association, and similar groups, are, of course, carefully controlled experiments utilizing purified vegetable oils and products known to be effective in lowering blood cholesterol. In order to make truly effective dietary recommendations, the public would have to be told what kinds and forms of vegetable oils to consume. Even if that were done, it's a safe bet that the manufacturers of products containing hydrogenated oils, coconut oil, etc. would continue advertising their products as being "cholesterol free"; "high in polyunsaturates", etc.

For that reason, the recommendations of the National Research Council appear to be the more prudent. Eat a balanced diet, and be careful to avoid overeating of any kind so as to maintain a bodyweight within normal ranges. Since overeating can increase blood cholesterol and triglycerides, and since obesity is itself a risk factor, people with normal metabolisms should be reasonably well protected if they follow this advice. If this advice is coupled with the American Medical Association's recommendation that everyone consult a physician and have a blood profile analysis run, the population as a whole would probably be as well protected as it could be. That is, by consulting a physician the people with abnormal cholesterol and triglyceride metabolisms could be identified and properly treated. Proper treatment, of course, may need

---

*A chemical process used to harden vegetable oils in the process of manufacturing vegetable shortening and margarine. That is, hardened in order that margarine may be made into "sticks"; vegetable shortening will have the consistency of lard for pie crusts, etc.

to include the use of drugs if diet alone is not sufficiently effective. Also, since dietary treatment may call for reduction of carbohydrates (instead of fats) in some instances, the people who really need specialized diets would be more certain of getting the diet they specifically need. Even if all the patient needs is a simple substitution of vegetable oils for saturated fats, it would be much better for him to receive the guidance of a knowledgeable dietitian since there are great differences in the ability of vegetable oil products to lower blood cholesterol levels.

Chapter 15 DIET, NUTRITION, AND CANCER

Cancer, of course, is probably the most insidious, frightening disease known to man. Its effect upon the body remains an enigma; the cause a mystery. Treatment consists of either removing (surgery) or killing (radiation, chemotherapy) the cancerous cells. There is some experimentation with a drug produced in the body as part of the immunity system (interferon), but the results have not been conclusive. Little more is known.

Most of what is known concerns the progression of the disease. As the Cancer Society has tried to impress upon us, if found in the early stages, most cancer can be cured. However, if left untreated, it essentially takes control of the body. The presence of a cancerous tumor is believed to cause the metabolism of the body to speed up (burn more energy). At the same time, cancer induces anorexia (loss of appetite). This causes the victim's body to emaciate, since more energy is being burned up, but less is being taken in. The diabolically strange thing about this situation is that while the body is deteriorating, the tumor can continue to grow. It has even been found that tumors can synthesize proteins. When the musculature is being broken down into its constituent amino acids, tumors can pull those amino acids out of the bloodstream, and synthesize them into proteins for their own growth.

Another fascinating but frightening aspect is that many cancerous tumors manufacture and release powerful drugs into the bloodstream. These drugs, many of them hormonal in nature, can have devastating effects upon the body. If left unchecked, death can either occur because of the metabolic changes created in the body, or the physical presence of the tumor blocks a vital function.

Because nearly everyone has watched someone close to them debilitated and destroyed by this physiological monster, there is great concern over its cause and prevention. Many people have expressed fear that compounds contained in the food supply may be carcinogenic. In general, these fears have been fueled by sensationalistic reporting of scientific research. However, while the dangers have often been exaggerated, there are some compounds that have carcinogenic potential.

NATURALLY OCCURRING CARCINOGENS IN THE FOOD SUPPLY

Avoiding foods that may have carcinogenic properties is no

simple matter. Practically every basic food staple has been implicated in one form of cancer or another. In some cases, foods that
appear to be linked to one type of cancer, also appear to be
protective of other forms of cancer. A list of foods that have been
linked would include:

Foodstuff	Type of Cancer
Fish (especially pickled and salted)	stomach
Cured and preserved meats	stomach
Polished rice	stomach
Leafy and green vegetables	stomach
Potatoes	stomach
Beans	stomach
Meat, animal fat	colon
Vegetable oil	breast and colon

Obviously, if one were to eliminate all the foods that have been
implicated, there would be very little left to eat. While it seems
ludicrous that all these foods could be harmful, when the incidence
of different types of cancer is analyzed internationally, the type
of diet eaten in each country is indicative of the type of
digestive tract cancer that will be most common.

For example, stomach cancer is the most common type of
digestive organ cancer. It has been associated with high fish
consumption, and as one might expect, countries such as Japan,
Iceland, and Finland have a very high incidence of stomach cancer
(approximately five times the rate of the US). [54] The agents thought
to be primarily responsible are the nitrosamines, which are known
to be powerful carcinogens. Nitrosamines are formed when compounds known as secondary amines come in contact with nitrates
and nitrites in an acid environment (as would be found in the
stomach). [55]

Fish is very high in secondary amines (amines are what give
fish its characteristic odor). Nitrates are found in green and leafy
vegetables,* cured meats,** and some water supplies. Pickled
or smoked fish is high in both nitrates and secondary amines.

*Plants absorb nitrogen through the roots in the form of nitrate, for synthesis
into proteins.
**Nitrites are added as a preservative.

Pickled vegetables (as are common in the Orient) are extremely high in nitrates. With this in mind, it is easy to see why the maritime nations have a very high incidence rate of stomach cancer. Studies conducted with the populations of Japan and Portugal, have shown that when immigrants have moved to the U.S., the rate of stomach cancer has declined for those people.[55]

Several of the Soviet Block nations also have very high rates of stomach cancer. (Czechoslovakia is reported to have the highest total cancer death rate in the world). These nations also consume substantial quantities of fish, especially dried and salted fish.* In addition, these countries also eat considerable amounts of cabbage (relatively high in nitrates), pickled vegetables, cured meats, and sausages.

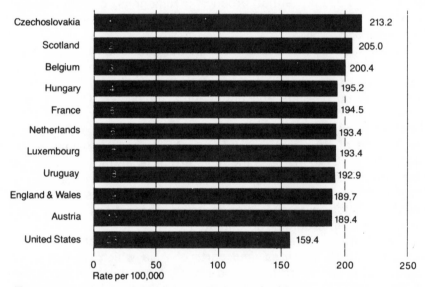

Figure 15-1. Cancer death rate for various countries.
Source: Cancer Facts and Statistics 1980, American Cancer Society.

Edible beans are quite high in nitrites, and have been implicated in stomach cancer. Possibly, beans may at least partially be responsible for the high rate of stomach cancer reported in the Latin American countries of Costa Rica, Chile, Guatamala, and Colombia.[54] Since these countries also border the sea, one could probably expect significant fish consumption as well.

*Provided by the Russian fishing fleet.

Other foods statistically implicated in stomach cancer include polished rice, and potatoes.[56] The actual mechanisms involved have not been clearly elucidated.

In the United States and western Europe, the stomach cancer rate is relatively low. Cancer of the colon, however, is relatively high. The foods linked to this type of cancer have been meat and fat (both animal and vegetable). An accentuating factor is thought to be the lack of fiber which characterizes Western diets.

The exact compounds or actions of meat and fats are not known at this time. Most of the theories center around action of the bacteria that inhabit the large intestine. It is believed that the bile acids secreted for fat digestion may be acted upon by the bacteria to form carcinogens. It has also be postulated that excess protein consumption, which results in putrefaction in the large intestine, may either produce carcinogens, or may change the type of bacteria present, which may themselves produce carcinogens.[54]

As mentioned, the lack of fiber in the U.S. and Western diets is thought to be an accentuating factor. Fiber (from vegetables, fruits, and whole grains) increases the amount of fecal matter, and speeds up passage and elimination. If bacterial action does indeed produce carcinogens from bile acids and proteins, then a lack of fiber would concentrate those compounds, and increase the amount of time they are in contact with the intestinal walls. Also, fiber tends to increase the moisture of fecal matter. Without fiber, the feces become dry and hard, which tends to irritate the colon (lack of fiber is thought to predispose the onset of diverticulitis). Thus, with the colon irritated, the actions of any carcinogens present would be accentuated.[57]

Cereal grains have been statistically linked with cancer of the liver. Countries in Africa, and parts of Asia which depend upon cereal grains as the primary food staple, have much higher rates of liver cancer than the more affluent nations. However, while there is a statistical link between cancer of the liver and cereal grains, the cause is not believed to be directly due to the grains themselves. Rather, the cause is believed to be due to aflatoxin formed by the mold Aspergillus flavus, which is well known to be a potent carcinogen.[54] In the developed countries where grain handling is mechanized and sophisticated, the development of molds is minimal, and likewise the incidence of liver cancer is very rare. In the underdeveloped nations the opposite is true.

In some scientific circles it is thought that the high incidence of kwashiorkor in underdeveloped nations may tend to predispose the liver to cancer, or accentuate the actions of aflotoxins.[54]

Kwashiorkor is a deficiency disease caused by a lack of balanced proteins in the diet, and is very common in nations which rely on cereal grains as the mainstay of the diet. One of the physiological effects upon the body is abnormal fat metabolism by the liver. Large amounts of fat are deposited at the liver, resulting in a bloated, pot-bellied look (Figure 15-2). It is believed that this may stress the liver and therefore make it more susceptible to cancer producing substances.

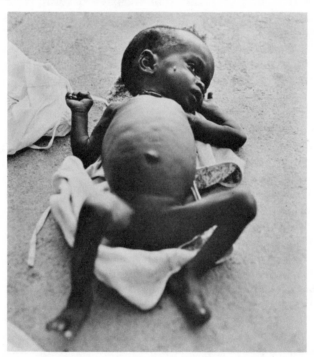

Figure 15-2. Child with Kwashiorkor. A disorder of malnutrition caused by a lack of balanced proteins in the diet. Large amounts of fat become deposited at the liver, which results in the enlarged appearance of the abdomen. Whether this is a factor in the high rate of liver cancer in peoples who subsist on cereal grains, it isn't known. (Photo courtesy of International Christian Aid, Los Angeles.)

In the final analysis, it would appear that there is nothing inherently cancerous about cereal grains, as long as they are free of molds, and are balanced with quality proteins.

The only foodstuff that has not been implicated in some type of cancer is fresh fruit. Indeed, several studies have shown fruit to be protective of stomach cancer.[58] One study, which examined Japanese immigrants in Hawaii, reported vitamin C (as contained in fruit) to be the protective factor. It is known that ascorbic acid (vitamin C) reacts with nitrite to render it incapable of combining with amines to form nitrosamines (the carcinogen associated with stomach cancer). It is therefore commonly accepted that this is the mode of action responsible for the reduced stomach cancer associated with fruit.

Care should be exercised in interpreting this. With apologies to the reader, it should be pointed out that there are those who would interpret this to mean that massive quantities of vitamin C are called for.* This is not true. What this means is that moderate levels of vitamin C (as are contained in fruit) would need to be consumed at the same time as the foods containing nitrites (vegetables, cured meats, etc.) and amines (fish, other protein foods). If the source of vitamin C is not present in the stomach at the same time as the nitrites and amines, it would not be effective. Therefore, taking a vitamin C tablet (once a day), would not be effective, regardless of the size of the dose.

It should also be pointed out that the fiber contained in fruit is very high in pectin. Pectin tends to absorb and hold water at a high rate, and is laxative. It would therefore seem reasonable to conclude that fruit could also be protective of cancer of the colon.

Conclusions on foodstuffs. From the previous discussion it seems obvious that dietary excesses should be avoided. People in maritime nations should make an effort to include fresh fruits in their diet, and substitute conventional meats and proteins for at least part of the fish in their diet (especially pickled or smoked fish). Fresh vegetables should be substituted for pickled vegetables.

People in the U.S. and western Europe should make an effort to include more fiber in their diet. Fruits and vegetables should be included with each meal, and whole grains substituted for highly processed carbohydrates (white flour and sugar). Excesses of proteins and fats should be avoided.

Moreover, all one need do is consume a balanced diet. While so many different food staples have been implicated, there really is no call for alarm. The fact of the matter is that digestive organ cancer in the U.S. and western Europe is not a major problem. As will be discussed later on in the chapter, lung cancer (as induced by cigarette smoking) is far and away the leading cause of cancer death. Indeed, while the total number of cancer deaths has been

*There are those who might even extrapolate this to mean that vitamin C is a cancer cure. This is not true, and isn't even logical.

increasing, the increase has almost entirely been due to lung cancer (Figure 15-5a & b).

NUTRITIONAL ASPECTS OF HORMONALLY INDUCED CANCERS

Breast cancer, cancer of the uterus, cervix, ovaries, prostate, and testis are deemed to be induced, or at least influenced by hormonal agents. While the nutritional aspects of digestive organ cancer (stomach, colon, and liver) appear reasonably clear, there is very little known about the nutritional aspects of hormonally related cancers.

Indeed, the only known link between hormonal cancer and anything . . . is uterine cancer and promiscuity. Statistical evaluations have indicated that multiple sex partners tends to be a predisposing factor. Prostitutes tend to have relatively high rates of uterine and vaginal cancer, whereas those types of cancer are practically unknown in Nuns.[56] (With respect to drugs, it is known that DES, a synthetic estrogen formerly used to prevent miscarriages, did cause higher incidences of vaginal cancer in daughters of the women consuming the drug).

With respect to foods, all that is known is that underfeeding tends to reduce the incidence of hormonal cancer, whereas overfeeding tends to increase it. Overnutrition and obesity are known to alter hormonal patterns, and obviously, this is thought to be at least part of the mechanism creating increased incidences of tumors.

Of the hormonal cancers, breast cancer has by far the greatest incidence rate, and consequently has been the most intensly studied. Asian and African countries have a low rate of incidence, whereas the affluent nations typically have a high rate of incidence. Comparing the diets of these diversly different areas and peoples, shows a statistical link with fat consumption.[59]

Research with laboratory animals has shown a greater incidence of breast cancer with the addition of fat to the diet, especially vegetable fat. Studies with corn oil have consistently shown a greater incidence rate than animal fats.[59] There are a number of theories to explain why vegetable oils would be more carcinogenic, but none are commonly accepted. Many authorities believe great care should be exercised in extrapolating this data to humans, since the natural diets of most laboratory animals are very low in fat.

Studies with human populations have been inconclusive. Some studies comparing the vegetable oil and animal fat intake of different groups have shown a higher rate of cancer for the groups eating more vegetable oil, but others have shown no difference. In one study, the women of Holland were compared to the women of Finland. Both groups eat approximately the same amount of animal fat, but the Dutch eat four times as much vegetable fat, and have twice the breast cancer rate. Studies with men put on low cholesterol, high polyunsaturated fat diets have in some instances shown a higher cancer death rate (than men on normal diets), and in other instances no difference, or a lower death rate. [58]

In relation to breast cancer (as well as other hormone related cancers), while there is a statistical link to fat, the relationship may be only coincidental. As some authorities point out, the actual mechanism involved may be calories (total caloric intake), rather than fat persay. As has been previously mentioned, when total caloric intake of laboratory animals is reduced, so also is the spontaneous development of cancerous tumors. The depression in intake however, must be severe . . . about a one-third reduction in what would ordinarily be considered an adequate intake. As at least one researcher has pointed out, this level of reduction would correspond to the subsistance level diets of Asia and Africa . . . where breast cancer rates are low.[59] The protective factor may very well be that Asian and African women remain thin all their lives, rather than what they eat.

This point seems particularly valid when it is considered that not all peoples with low breast cancer rates consume low fat diets. As mentioned on p. 102, the pastoral tribes of East Africa consume diets extremely high in fat . . . living primarily off the cattle they herd. As most everyone has seen in National Geographic, or various television documentaries, the mainstay of their diet consists of a mixture of blood and milk, made into a form of porridge. (The cattle are routinely bled from the jugular vein, and the blood is then mixed with fresh milk.) This type of diet constitutes the highest fat intake in the world.[29] But while the amount of fat in the diet is very high, the total amount of calories is very low. The women therefore remain very thin all their lives (Figure 15-3). Obviously then, it may be the fact that they remain thin, rather than what they eat, that protects them from breast cancer   .

With respect to the amount of body fat, it is known that adipose tissue (fat tissue) can secrete hormones. This is particularly true after menapause. Estrogens, of course, are the primary female hormones. The term estrogens, however, is a catch-all term used to cover three distinct types of estrogen; E_1, known

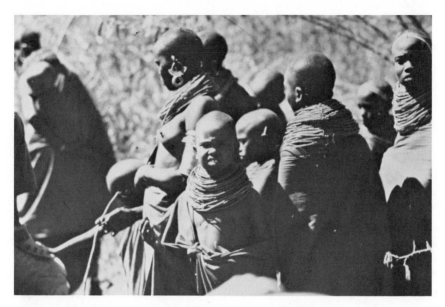

Figure 15-3. Women of the Samburu District in Kenya. Breast cancer rates in most third world countries are low. Since the diets in most of these nations are typically very low in fat, a statistical analysis would indicate fat as a factor. However, some primitive peoples such as these Samburu women, eat diets extremely high in fat (consisting primarily of cattle blood and milk). But while fat in the diet is very high, the total amount of calories is very low. What protects them from breast cancer may be the fact that they remain thin all their lives.

as estrone; E_2, known as estradiol; and E_3, known as estriol. After menapause, most women have higher levels of estrone, as this is the estrogen produced in greatest quantity by fatty tissues. Correspondingly, the risk of breast cancer increases substantially after menapause. At least one report has stated that obese women tend to have higher levels of estrone than slender women.[59]

Studies attempting to correlate obesity with breast cancer, however, have been inconclusive. Some authorities now postulate that nutrition (and obesity) at the time of menarch (onset of menstruation) may be more important than at the time breast cancer actually appears.[54,59] There is data to indicate that girls who reach menarch earlier, tend to have higher rates of breast cancer. While genetics is involved in the timing of menarch, it is also believed that nutrition may affect the age at which menstruation begins. The thought being that menarch is triggered more by height and weight than age. The level of nutrition, of course, would greatly influence height and weight.

Still, as mentioned at the beginning of this section, there is very little known. It does seem clear, however, that there are environmental differences that are affecting the incidences of breast cancer. For example, a study of Japanese women living in San Francisco showed them to have a substantially higher breast cancer rate than on the Japanese mainland. Studies with Japanese women in Hawaii, have shown them to have hormonal patterns more similar to caucasion women than Japanese nationals.[59]

Quite obviously, the answers have not been found. In addition to diet and nutrition, there could very well be other factors involved. For example, Dr. Otto Schaefer, a medical researcher in the Canadian Arctic, pointed out that breast cancer in Eskimo women living the traditional lifestyle is very low, but increases substantially when Eskimos "move to town".[60] Dr. Schaefer made the observation that when Eskimos accept Western lifestyles, they cease nursing their babies, and begin bottle feeding . . . and mentioned that this might be a factor. Dr. Schaefer

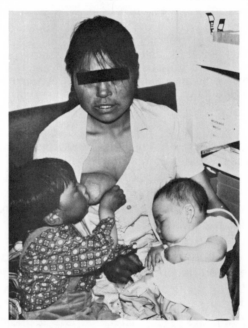

Figure 15-4. Dr. Otto Schaefer, a Canadian medical researcher reported greatly reduced breast cancer rates in Eskimo women living in their natural environment. Among the differences between "civilized" Eskimos and those living the traditional life is nursing. Traditional Eskimos breast feed their babies, whereas Eskimos "moved to town" often do not. Photo courtesy Dr. Otto Schaefer.

has also pointed out, however, that this change in lifestyle also includes an enormous change in diet; from a diet consisting primarily of animal protein and fish, to a typical western diet which includes substantial amounts of highly refined carbohydrates and vegetable fats, in addition to animal fats.[46] Probably equally (if not more) important, overeating and obesity become a factor as well.

In summary, there is very little that can be said in relation to preventing breast cancer and the other hormonally related cancers. Nutritionally, about the only thing that can be said is to avoid overeating. It would probably be wise to avoid overeating during adolescence as well as adult life. The kind of dietary restrictions that are endured by Asian and African peoples (and are known to be protective in laboratory animals) are not practical, and possibly injurious to health in general.

While there is very little understood concerning the cause of these diseases, it should be pointed out that substantial progress has been made in the treatment. Therefore, while the idea of some type of special diet may seem more appealing, the best advice is probably to have frequent check-ups so that if a neoplasm does develop, it can be removed or treated before it becomes life threatening. The only real dietary advice that can be offered at this time is to avoid excesses and maintain proper weight control.

FOOD ADDITIVES AND CANCER

In addition to the potential carcinogens which may occur naturally in food, many people are of the opinion that man-made additives may also pose a threat. At the present time, this is an issue of great controversy.

As a matter of official public health policy, it can be said that no man-made substance known to be capable of inducing cancer is contained in the food supply. This is due to what has come to be known as the Delaney Clause. In 1958 Congress ammended the Pure Food and Drug Act, which directed the FDA to totally ban any substance known to cause cancer. The Delaney Clause specified that the substance was to be banned if it caused cancer in man or animals, regardless of the concentration.

Because the Delaney Clause ignored the question of concentration, it has come to be very controversial. As the reader is probably aware, standard procedure for the testing of compounds involves feeding them to laboratory animals at many thousands (sometimes hundreds of thousands) of times the level they would ever be consumed by humans.

Critics of this type of testing contend that it is not realistic. They contend that some compounds may be entirely safe when consumed at their intended levels, but dangerous when consumed at the incredibly high levels used in testing. They also point out that the type of exposure the test animals are subjected to, is sometimes totally different than the way humans come in contact with the substance. For example, a hair dye product that was recently banned . . . was fed to the animals tested.

In addition to the amount and manner in which compounds are tested, there has also been criticism of the type of animal used. Over the last 15 to 20 years, special breeds of mice have been developed which are much more prone to develop cancer. These mice, which are capable of spontaneously developing tumors are the ones typically used in the testing of food additives.

Defenders of the present policy state that it is financially infeasible to test compounds any other way. They maintain that while human exposure to potential carcinogens may be small, the total impact may be substantial. For example, a carcinogen may cause one tumor out of every 10,000 people exposed to it. With a population of 220 million, this could produce 22,000 cancers - a very serious situation.

The National Cancer Institute states that there is no feasible way they could test a compound at a level that would produce cancer in one out of every 10,000 mice. Because of the laws of chance, they would need tens of thousands of mice to do that. Obviously, feeding, housing, and examining 40 or 50 thousand mice would be enormously expensive. The Cancer Institute maintains that the only logistically feasible way is to take about 50 mice, and feed inordinately high levels of the compounds to be tested. In that way, if 20 or 30 of the mice come up with cancer, there is a good indication that the compound is indeed cancerous. Likewise, if high doses don't cause cancer, there is a much better chance the chemical is not a carcinogen.

In short, defenders of the present policy contend that no one can be sure if a carcinogen can have a "safe" level. Their belief is that when there is a low dosage level, there will be a low incidence rate of cancer.

Gras substances. Prior to enactment of the Pure Food and Drug Act of 1958, there were a large number of food additives already in use. Because these compounds had been in use for a number of years without any apparent problem, they were considered "Generally Recognized As Safe" (GRAS). It was felt that the FDA's resources would be better spent looking at new compounds, about which nothing was known.

Before 1958, prior approval was not required to use food additives. After 1958, any new food additive had to be submitted to the FDA before it could be used.

The GRAS substances are periodically reviewed, and if any question arises concerning a substance, the FDA tests it. In all, about 250 have been tested, and several have been banned (the most well known having been the artificial sweeteners cyclamate and saccarin, and red dye #2).

TYPES OF ADDITIVES

There are two basic types of additives; intentional, and unintentional. Intentional additives would include artificial colors, flavors, flavor enhancers, preservatives, as well as synthetic vitamins and mineral supplements. Unintentional additives include trace amounts of packaging materials, pesticides, herbicides, antibiotics and drugs used in livestock. All of these compounds fall under the Delaney Clause of the Pure Food and Drug Act.

Pesticides. Pesticides and other agricultural chemicals probably cause people more concern than any other compounds known to be in the food supply. Quite obviously, they are certainly toxic compounds. However, it should be understood that a compound may be toxic, but not carcinogenic. There are several thousand compounds known to be toxic, but there are only about 30 compounds known to be carcinogenic.[61]

One should also understand that the amounts of pesticides and other agricultural chemicals found in food, are present only in infinitesimally small amounts. Likewise, it should also be realized that animals and humans can tolerate a number of toxic compounds without ill effect, when the daily dosage level is low. For example, there are a very large number of naturally occurring toxic substances that we consume every day. Potatoes contain solanine, a highly toxic substance when concentrated; turnips and onions contain alkaloids that can cause rupture of the red blood cells when concentrated; lima beans contain hydrogen-cyanide; salt water fish typically contain arsenic and mercury. The list could go on and on.

Pesticides are the most regulated compounds in the food supply.

Before a pesticide can be approved for use, a need must exist for the product, and it must be proved to be effective for that purpose. It must then be determined what the maximum residual level on a crop would be.* The Product is then fed to no less than two animal species at levels of 100 to 1000 times the maximum residue level. During this testing if it is found to be harmful, the product will not be cleared for use. However, even if it is not found to be harmful at these levels, it can still be banned if found to cause cancer at any level. That is, if fed at hundreds of thousands of times the residue level, the product causes cancer . . . it is banned.

Drugs used in livestock. In some instances, meat, eggs, and poultry contain trace amounts of drugs used in the animal. In most cases, after administering a drug, a withdrawal period is required before the animals may be slaughtered, or eggs, milk, etc., may be kept for human consumption. The withdrawal period is designed to bring residues in the animal or food product down to a zero, or near zero trace level.

Again, the Delaney Clause is very much in effect. For example, during the 1960's and 70's, DES, a synthetic hormone was widely used in women to prevent miscarriage. It was also used as a growth promotant in beef cattle. When it was discovered that daughters of women who took DES had a greater likelihood of developing vaginal cancer, the use of DES in animals was banned. Residues had never been found in the meat. The only residues ever found were in the liver, at levels of only 1 or 2 parts per million (in less than one tenth of one percent of the animals slaughtered). It was pointed out that a woman would have to eat several thousand pounds of liver, just to get the same amount of DES contained in one "morning after" birth control pill (another use of the drug). Still, the ban was upheld. With respect

---

*There are, of course, the so-called organically grown foods without pesticides. To begin with, because there is no way to tell "organically" grown food from ordinary crops, fraud has been commonplace.

In order to legitimately produce organic crops, they must be grown well away from established agricultural areas (crop pests). Even in isolated areas, however, one would expect damaging insects and other pests to arrive within two or three seasons, forcing movement of the operation. Moreover, there is potential for feeding only a small fraction of the population with organically grown food.

Our only hope in this area is research into what is known as biological control. That is, the use of other insects, birds, etc. to control crop pests.

to carcinogenity, there is no flexibility.*

INTENTIONAL ADDITIVES

There are currently over 3000 food additives in use today. A majority of these compounds were in use before 1958, and are therefore considered GRAS (Generally Recognized as Safe). Because only about 250 of these compounds have been thoroughly tested, some people have questions about the safety of prepared foods.

However, experts in the field of public health rate food additives as one of the lowest risk areas. [62, 56] With respect to cancer, the information that is available would indicate that they are right. Cancer death rates have been going up, but the increase has been primarily due to one type of cancer . . . lung cancer (Figure 15-5a & b). Stomach cancer in the U.S. has declined by over 60%. Liver cancer is very rare. If there were indeed a number of cancerous food additives, one would expect a relatively high level of liver cancer. The function of the liver is to filter toxic substances out of the blood, and it would seem logical to conclude that cancerous substances in food would tend to increase liver cancer.

SUMMARY AND CONCLUSIONS ON FOOD ADDITIVES

There are a large number of additives contained in the food supply; many of them intentional; some of them unintentional. For the most part, the unintentional additives (pesticides, and animal drugs) have undergone intensive testing and evaluation. Their presence in the food supply is tolerated only at infinitesimally minute levels.

Intentional additives are present in much larger quantities. In addition, because the great majority of these compounds (artificial colors and flavors, flavor enhancers, preservatives, etc.) were in use before the Pure Food and Drug Act of 1958, only a fraction of them have been subjected to the intensive type of testing described previously. This is what causes many people concern. As discussed, the indication is that food additives

*With respect to non-carcinogenic toxicity in humans, the rules are also quite strict. If a drug is known to cause severe reactions in humans, it may not be used in livestock. There are a number of veterinary medicines cleared for use in horses, dogs, and other pets, but not food animals. The reason being that they cause either toxicity or allergic reactions in humans.

provide minimum cancer risk. Still, it seems significant that every few years the FDA identifies one of the GRAS substances (pre-1958 additives) as being a potential carcinogen. Because of this, it would seem prudent to avoid food additives whenever possible. Quite clearly, the majority of the food additives have no nutritional value, only cosmetic or commercial value. Therefore there can certainly be no harm in avoiding artificially colored or flavored foods. Indeed, since many of these products are associated with what are commonly termed "junk foods", there may be some nutritional advantage.

TOBACCO AND ALCOHOL

Most people know that cigarette smoking contributes to lung cancer, heart disease, and a few other diseases and disorders. However, only a relatively few people realize the extent of the damage cigarettes can do, and the magnitude of the danger they represent.

If it were not for cigarette smoking, the cancer death rate would be declining. Looking at Figure 15-5a & b, one can see the rapid increase in lung cancer over the last 40 years. Eighty percent of all lung cancer deaths are attributable to smoking.[56]

While most people are aware of smoking and its relation to lung cancer, few people are aware of the contribution smoking makes to other cancers. Smoking is known to be a significant factor in cancer of the bladder,* pancreas, esophagus, larynx (voicebox), throat, and mouth. In addition, smoking greatly magnifies the effect industrial carcinogens have on an individual. For example, the American Cancer Society has calculated that an asbestos worker who smokes increases his cancer risk over 90 times that of a worker who doesn't smoke.[63]

Probably one of the reasons the warnings on cigarettes have not been effective is the fact that lung cancer takes a long time to develop. There is a time lag of some 15 to 20 years. Looking at Figures 15-5a & b we can see when smoking became popular. Among men, widespread smoking began during World War I. Correspondingly, lung cancer rates began to accelerate after 1935. Smoking among women did not begin until the 1940's. Up until that time it was considered unladylike. World War II and the mobilization of women into the labor

---

*Smokers have 2 to 3 times the chance of developing cancer of the bladder.

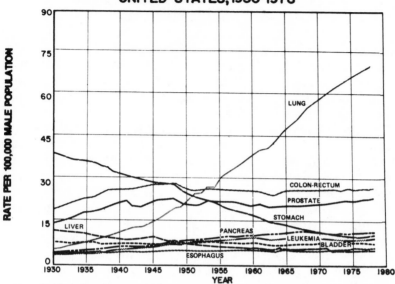

MALE CANCER DEATH RATES BY SITE
UNITED STATES, 1930-1978

Figure 15-5a & b. Cancer death rates in the U.S. have been increasing, but only due to one type of cancer . . . lung cancer. If it weren't for cigarette smoking, the cancer death rate might actually begin to decline.
Source: 1982 Cancer Facts and Statistics, American Cancer Society.

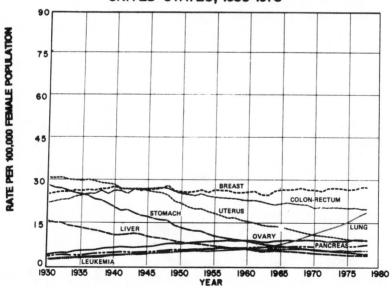

FEMALE CANCER DEATH RATES BY SITE
UNITED STATES, 1930-1978

force changed all that. Working on the assembly lines and in the shipyards broke a lot of taboos, and the new "liberated" women of this country were free to smoke. Smoke they did . . . and as can be seen in Figure 15-5b, beginning about 1965 they began to pay for it. As the reader can see, the slope of the lung cancer curve for women beginning in 1965 is essentially identical to the one for men beginning in 1935. It seems reasonable to conclude that the lung cancer curve for women will continue an upward path similar to the one for men.

The use of alcohol intensifies the effects of tobacco in oral cancers. As discussed in Chap. 9, alcohol is known to dissolve the protective lining of the stomach and small intestine. Most likely, the same type of action is responsible for the increased risk of oral cancer. That is, alcohol irritates the lining of the mouth, throat, and esophagus, and thereby makes the tissue more susceptible to the action of tobacco (either as smoke, or as chewing tobacco). Survival of oral cancers is much better than lung cancer. Only about 10% of the people with lung cancer survive more than 5 years after first diagnosis, whereas the survival rate with oral cancer is about 50%.[63] However, when oral cancer is survived, there are often very deep emotional/personality problems to deal with. Surgery of the lips, cheeks, and gums often leaves a frightening disfigurement, and surgery on the larynx usually leaves one unable to communicate except by what is known as esophageal speech (forming words with swallowed air). Ironically, smoking typically begins during adolescence as a means of looking sophisticated.

The real tragedy among tobacco and alcohol related cancers, of course, is that it is so unnecessary . . . so easily preventable. Quitting smoking, of course, takes great discipline. But like everything else in life, there is very little that is worth obtaining, that doesn't carry a substantial price tag in terms of commitment. Likewise, quitting alcohol takes great courage . . . courage to face life as it is, or in the case of our youth, courage to face peer pressure with strength of personal conviction.

SUMMARY OF THE NUTRITIONAL ASPECTS OF CANCER

Most of the public's concern over carcinogens in the food supply centers around the use of man-made additives. However, the cancers known to be caused by substances in the food supply, are primarily naturally occurring compounds.

Stomach cancer, the most common type of digestive organ

cancer, is well known to be caused by nitrosamines. Diets high in fish and pickled vegetables are clearly implicated in stomach cancer (compounds in fish and vegetables combine to form nitrosamines). Diets excessively high in meat and fat, but low in fiber, are believed to be implicated in cancer of the colon.

Research work with laboratory animals has indicated that hormonally related cancers may be linked with overeating, and/or excessive fat consumption. In relation to breast cancer, there is some indication that overeating during adolescence may be as important as after menapause (when most breast cancer actually occurs).

Probably the best dietary advice that can be given is to eat balanced meals, and avoid dietary excesses. Inclusion of fresh fruit during meals would do much to prevent stomach cancer, and the inclusion of both fruit, and fresh vegetables would do much to prevent cancer of the colon. Likewise, substitution of whole cereal grains for refined carbohydrates (flour, sugar, etc.) would probably be protective of cancer of the colon. Excesses of proteins and fats should be avoided.

Tobacco is still far and away the leading cause of cancer death. Indeed, the cancer death rate in the U.S. would be declining, if it were not for lung cancer. In addition to lung cancer, tobacco is known to be a major factor in cancer of the bladder, pancreas, and the oral cancers. The effect of industrial carcinogens is known to be enormously affected by cigarette smoke.

Ultimately, it should be remembered that early detection of tumors is of vital importance for survival. The nutritional aspects of cancer may be of moderate importance, but it is no substitute for frequent examinations. Everyone should learn the warning signals of cancer* and seek prompt examination should any of them occur.

*Change in bowel or bladder habits.
 A sore that does not heal.
 Unusual bleeding or discharge.
 Thickening or lump in breast or elsewhere.
 Indigestion or difficulty in swallowing.
 Obvious change in wart or mole.
 Nagging cough or hoarseness.

Chapter 16   DIVERTICULITIS (Inflamed Bowel) AND CONSTIPATION

Diverticulitis and constipation are disorders considered to be unique to affluent nations. In the third world countries these problems are virtually unknown.

Differences in diet, and to a lesser extent, physical activity, are said to be responsible. The diet in most underdeveloped nations is typically high in whole cereal grains, beans, roots, and tubers. All of these foods are high in fiber.

The diet consumed in most affluent nations is very low in fiber. The carbohydrate fraction of the diet consisting primarily of processed white flour and sugar. White flour, of course, does not contain the bran or the germ of the grain - only the starch. Therefore, flour is very low in fiber. Sugar contains no fiber.

Dietary fiber absorbs water and therefore makes the stool softer. A diet low in fiber produces a smaller, much harder stool. It is believed that this type of stool tends to irritate and inflame the colon. Therefore, it is often recommended that persons suffering from diverticulitis consume a diet high in fiber.

The high fiber diet helps in several ways. First of all, since high fiber stools are softer and more watery, there is less physical abrasion. Secondly, because there is more volume to the stool, chemical irritants such as bile acids are diluted, and therefore are not able to irritate the colonic membranes like they could in a more concentrated form. Also, high fiber tends to speed up passage through the digestive tract, which limits the time chemical irritants are in contact with the walls of the colon.[65] These same functions of fiber are also thought to be protective of cancer of the colon (p. 116).

Lack of physical exercise, in addition to low fiber diets is thought to be a predisposing factor in constipation. For most people, a moderate daily exercise program, and inclusion of some fruit, vegetables, or whole grain with each meal will eliminate problems with constipation.

The situation with diverticulitis is not quite as clear as with constipation. However, it does seem that exercise and a moderate amount of fiber in the diet are protective. Diets extremely high in fiber should not be undertaken except under the direction of a physician. Likewise, people already suffering any kind of intestinal problem should not make any substantial dietary changes without consulting a physician.

SECTION III - REFERENCE

Chapter 17   LOW CALORIE COOKING
By Cheryl Price

To many people, the idea of low calorie dishes conjures up the idea of tasteless, bland foods. This needn't be the case. In fact, most of our own favorite recipes can be modified to greatly reduce calories, while at the same time increasing flavor.

A large percentage of our dessert recipes can be easily modified to reduce sugar and/or increase fiber. Some main course items can also be modified in this manner, especially if the item is home-made vs. commercially prepared. If done gradually, these modifications will barely be missed, but once the transition is completed, using the original recipe will be very noticeable. You'll be amazed at how sickening sweet things you've always eaten will taste once you're accustomed to more flavor and less sweet.

To achieve this change start with small changes and obvious over uses. Some examples would be; changing from using milk chocolate chips to semisweet chips in cookies, etc. It's a small caloric saving, but it will accustom your taste for less sugar. Rinse the sugar crystals from chopped dates before including them as an ingredient. Use fruit canned in lite syrups and/or rinse canned fruit with water before serving. Buy "natural" or unsweetened applesauce for use plain or as an ingredient. Jam made with ½ the normal sugar is also a good place to start cutting back, and can be carried further by using unsweetened fruit puree.

Dessert items, of course, usually contain the highest level of sugar (as unnecessary calories). In nearly all recipes, sugar can usually be cut in at least half. In many cases, one third to one fourth the amount of sugar called for will usually suffice. This is particularly true for items that contain fruit, or nuts. The natural sweetness, of course, adds to the sweetness of the recipe, but the natural flavor is also a contributory factor. By cutting down on the added sugar, the true flavor of the recipe is allowed to come through. By substituting more of the main ingredients (fruits, etc.) for much of the sugar, you will indeed have a more flavorful recipe. Commercially prepared desserts typically are just the opposite - they add extra amounts of sugar and/or corn syrup as a partial substitute for the much more expensive items in the product (cherries, pecans, etc.). The idea being that the sweet taste will override the reduced amount of main ingredient.

Pies, custards, etc. that use sugar as a thickening agent are more difficult to modify. However, in many cases adding extra eggs to the recipe will help achieve the desired consistency. For items such as pecan or pumpkin pie, a great deal of the sugar can be reduced if an extra egg is added to the filling mix.

Obviously, pies with only one crust substantially cut down the amount of carbohydrate by eliminating the top crust. Further reduction can be accomplished by using whole wheat flour in the crust recipe. Because whole wheat flour contains considerable fiber and oil (from the wheat germ), it does not hold together as well as bleached, refined flour. As a result, pie crusts made with whole wheat flour tend to tear much more easily. Experimentation will teach just how much whole wheat can be substituted.

The caloric content of graham cracker crusts can be greatly reduced by eliminating all the additional sugar called for. Graham crackers are sweet by themselves, and sugar is certainly not needed when they are used as a crust, especially under a sweet pie filling. This same ommission would apply to other dessert crusts such as mud pie, bar cookies, etc.

Cakes are also targets for cutting back on layers of sweetness. When the cake is sweet, use a plain icing such as cream cheese. In reverse, if a sugary icing is being used, cut way back on the cake's sugar content. (For example, pineapple upside down cake with its sugar coating doesn't require any sugar in the cake.) Leaving the icing out between cake layers and substituting fruit filling, or other unsweetened fillings is another easy reduction. Instead of drizzling sugar glaze over a cake use fruit purees. (This can also apply to rolls and buns.) "Pudding cakes" (commercial cake and pudding mixes combined) also combine the sugar of two desserts. Use a scratch cake recipe omitting the sugar, and the commercial pudding mix, or use the commercial cake mix with sour cream or yogurt as the moistening agent.

Other desserts often call for these double doses of sugar. Its just a matter of being aware of them as they can usually be easily reduced. For example, bar cookies will call for milk chocolate, marshmellows, corn syrup, etc. Unsweetened chocolate or carob is the easiest cut. Secondly, the corn syrup could probably be reduced or substituted in accordance with the remainder of the recipe.

Applesauce cake, date bread, banana bread, etc. which are sweetened by other ingredients can eventually have all sugar omitted. This allows the flavor of the other ingredients to come through much stronger. Actually increasing the "name" ingredient (bananas, carrots, squash, etc.) can benefit the bread/cake in flavor and nutrition. Depending on the ingredient, fiber, vitamins, and minerals will be increased. Also, physical properties like moistness is usually enhanced.

Trying for flavor as opposed to sweetness is also applicable to cookies. Cut back on sugar but increase nuts, spices, fruit, extracts, etc. Textures can also replace sweetness for variety; that is crunchy, creamy, etc.

Dessert toppings. Whipped cream is, of course, a very high calorie food item due to the high butterfat content. Many of us trying to cut calories simply omit cream as a topping on desserts, but some dishes require whipped cream as an ingredient or essential part of the recipe. Most of these desserts are sweet in themselves and the tablespoon or two of sugar beaten into the cream is the first thing to omit in reducing the calories. A more drastic caloric reduction can be achieved by substituting a very thick powdered non-fat milk mix for the cream. Use equal parts of icy water and powdered milk (about ½ cup each to top 4 desserts) and beat together. This will take more beating than cream to create a peaked topping. (Partially freezing the mix will cut the whipping time.) Also, the stiffness will not last as long, but the mix can be rebeaten. If it is necessary for the peaks to last longer, add a bit more powdered milk. Instead of adding sugar to whipped toppings, try different flavorings such as almond, vanilla, mint, etc.

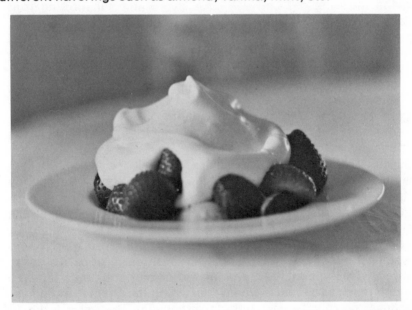

Figure 17-1. Equal parts of ice water and powdered milk can be beaten to form an excellent low calorie dessert topping. Not only is it much lower in calories than whipped cream or commercial toppings, but it is much more nutritious. For variety, try adding flavorings such as almond, vanilla, mint, etc. (instead of sugar).

Egg whites can also be used as a whipped ingredient substitute, either as the traditional meringue topping, or as a volume increasing ingredient. They can be whipped and folded just as cream would be, although they will not hold their volume indefinitely, unless baked. As with powdered milk toppings, egg whites can be mixed with flavor extracts for variety.

Gelatin. Although used as a meal accompaniment, gelatin salads are also in the dessert class. Those salads made with fruit, marsh-mallows, etc. can be made with plain gelatin and fruit juice instead. of commercial flavored gelatins which contain sugar.

Use of yogurt, cottage cheese, or sour cream. Equal amounts of yogurt, sour cream, or cottage cheese are often interchangeable. Sour cream is the most caloric, but also has the smoothest taste, and is the creamiest. Yogurt (plain) has the least number of calo-ries, but the natural unsweetened variety has an acid taste to over-come. In breads and cakes this is not usually a problem, as their sweetness and flavors mask the yogurt. Baking also does much to overcome the acid flavor. Even when substituting yogurt for sour cream, most recipes can take a 50% sugar reduction with-out the sharp flavor coming through. If commercially made yogurt is used, even more sugar may be omitted as most brands contain a sweetener. Sour cream and cottage cheese do not have this sharp taste and therefore they too will work with a lower sugar level. Low fat, small curd cottage cheese can be utilized to add moistness to breads, cakes, etc. also. For a creamier. texture, run cottage cheese through a blender to create a puree. While not quite as smooth as sour cream, it is lower in fat.

These substitutions are also applicable for dressings. Even using sour cream instead of mayonaise with powdered dressing mixes creates a substantial reduction in calories, and the tang of yogurt is not unwelcome in salad dressing. Chef salads or other green salads can go without dressing if tossed with cottage cheese plus some seasoning such as lemon juice, paprika, etc. Toss fruit salads with yogurt or sour cream in place of mayonaise for a change (the oil in mayonaise gives it a much higher calorie content).

As mentioned in chapter 6, commercially produced yogurt generally has some type of sweetener added to it, especially the fruit flavors. Making your own yogurt gives you the option of varying the ingredients to suit your use. When using plain yogurt in items like dressings, breads, etc., all sweeteners can be omitted. As a dessert in itself, try using just fruit puree, or sauces without additional sugar. Unsweetened applesauce blended with yogurt makes a good dessert sauce. For variety, try using pureed baby fruits, as opposed to canned fruits as most of the baby fruits do not have added sugar.

To obtain a firmer consistancy (similar to commercial varieties) when making yogurt at home, dissolve a packet of unflavored gelatin (per quart of milk) when pre-boiling the milk. The yogurt will be thin when incubating, but upon refrigeration will set up.

Whole wheat flour. Whole wheat flour contains the bran and germ of the grain and therefore is nutritionally a better choice than white flour. Unfortunately, it has aspects we are not used to. Its flavor is not as bland as white flour and can cause a somewhat bitter taste in delicately flavored foods. The coarser texture also presents some problems when used in pie crusts, pastries, and cakes, etc., as it imparts a tendency to crumble or tear.

To cope with these differences in recipes which call for white flour, it is best to make the change gradually. Trial and error will eventually give you an adaptation that works . . . but to start with, try a mixture of ½ white and ½ whole wheat flour for most baked goods. From there you can go "forward" or "backward" depending on the resultant flavor and/or texture. If texture is the limiting factor, the amount you substitute will be a matter of your personal preference.

Fortunately, in most cases it is only the flavor that regulates the use of whole wheat flour. When this is the case, gradually decrease the amount of white flour (while increasing the whole wheat), as you gradually decrease sugar in both your diet and recipes. Also, as mentioned in the section on decreasing sugar, use other flavors to overcome blandness. Just as fruits, extracts, etc. can substitute for the sweet taste, they can also overcome the mildly bitter whole wheat taste.

When flour (or corn starch) is used as a thickening agent in gravies, sauces, puddings, etc., the same rule applies. (It's rare that texture is a problem in these instances.) Gradually substitute whole wheat flour and perhaps put extra cheese in the cheese sauce or another banana in the pudding, etc.

One caution that should increase your chances of following through on converting your recipes, is to avoid doing it all at once. Don't try to cut back the sugar and increase the whole wheat flour on the first recipe change. First cut down on the sugar. When you've adjusted to that, then substitute some whole wheat flour. In this way you can live with the changes, and come to enjoy them, rather than suffer through them.

Bran can be added to many recipes that call for flour and some which don't. Bran can create the same problems as whole wheat flour, and its addition should be approached in the same manner. If you have otherwise altered your diet by including more fruit and vegetables, whole grains, and substituting a portion of whole wheat flour for white, the addition of bran is probably not necessary.

Bran, of course, is nothing more than the outer seed coat of wheat, and is therefore contained in whole wheat flour. Rather than simply adding bran to white flour, it is probably best to add whole wheat flour, as in most cases it will be a coarser texture than white flour. Coarser texture means it cannot be digested as rapidly, and in most cases is therefore less fattening.

Foods other than desserts and pastries. Meals can be made more nutritious and less caloric by using the same substitutions described in the previous sections. Many courses besides dessert call for sugar or sweeteners that are unnecessary.

Obviously those pinches of sugar put in vegetables can be dropped. There are several options for dressing up yams and sweet potatoes besides marshmallows. Sour cream thinned with milk is a more nutritious option.

Tomato based sauces like spagetti sauce and bar-b-que sauce often contain sugar. Most of these recipes can be changed to exclude sugar without any other adjustments. Some such as home-made bar-b-que sauce call for ketchup and additional sugar. Since ketchup is about 30% sweeteners, the additional sugar will not be missed from the sauce.

Sweet and sour sauce, used on a variety of entrees, can probably be juggled to cut back its sugar content. One recipe, as an example, called for 1 cup each of sugar, vinegar, and pineapple juice as the major ingredients. Using only ½ cup each of the sugar and vinegar, but increasing the pineapple juice to 1½ cups gives excellent results.

When making gravies, it is relatively easy to remove most of the fat while retaining most of the natural juices (with most meats, the juices will contain the highest concentration of the B vitamins). There are essentially two ways to do this. The old fashioned way would be to stir ice cubes around in the warm gravy. The ice causes the fat to congeal around the cubes, and can therefore be removed rather easily.

An even easier way to remove fat is with the new type of fat removing pitchers available. As you can see in figure 17-2, these pitchers have the pouring spout at the bottom of the cup. The fat being lighter, floats on the top - allowing you to pour off the juices (and water soluble vitamins) from the bottom.

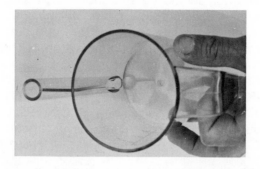

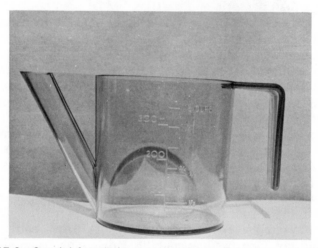

Figure 17-2. Special fat pitchers currently available are an excellent way to retain the cooking juices from meat, while pouring off the fat (the cooking juices, of course, contain much of the water soluble vitamins). These pitchers actually pour from the bottom. Thus, the fat floats on top, allowing you to easily separate the true juices from the fat.

Summary. Low calorie cooking is more a matter of adjusting your taste preferences than anything else. Because commercial products typically use heavy amounts of sugar to cover up other ingredients (or a lack of ingredients), most of us have become accustomed to very sweet foods. Therefore, when cutting down on sugar, don't try and do it all at once. The same goes for the substitution of whole wheat flour. Take it a step at a time, and let your family get used to it. Once you get used to more flavor and less sweet, you won't want to go back to your old recipes. Cherry pie, cobbler, etc., with two or three times as many cherries, really does taste better than a big load of sugar.

Chapter 18   VITAMINS

Vitamins are divided into two different categories; 1. fat soluble and; 2. water soluble. The fat soluble vitamins include vitamins A, D, E, and K. The water soluble vitamins are comprised of vitamin C, and all the B vitamins; Thiamine, Riboflavin, Pantothenic Acid, Biotin, Pyroxidine (B_6), Folacin, and Cobalamin (B_{12}).

The fat soluble vitamins can be stored in the body fat (and in some cases the liver). As a result, there isn't a pressing need for a daily intake of them. When daily intake is inadequate, the stored reserves can be used until intake is again adequate. Likewise, when more than enough is taken in on a given day, part of the excess is stored for future use.

Because the fat soluble vitamins can be stored, there is a much greater danger of toxicity. With water soluble vitamins, excessive quantities are usually just passed out with the urine. Massive doses can cause some problems within the digestive tract, but as a general rule, the kidney can filter excessive levels out of the blood. This is not the case with fat soluble vitamins. Toxicities can and have occurred with the fat soluble vitamins. Toxicities can occur either from massive short term doses, or excessive long term doses.

When vitamins are not consumed in sufficient amounts, deficiency symptoms occur. In most situations, adequate vitamin nutrition will reverse deficiency symptoms. As a practical matter, vitamin deficiencies do not occur in healthy people when a balanced diet is eaten. Simple vitamin deficiencies occur primarily in underdeveloped countries where cereal grains or rice are the mainstay of the diet. In the industrialized nations, when vitamin deficiencies occur, it usually is due to induced malnutrition such as vegetarianism, or metabolic disturbances. Diseases which adversely affect digestion, can induce vitamin deficiencies. Anything that hinders fat digestion can reduce absorption of the fat soluble vitamins. Diseases that affect the gall bladder, pancreas, or liver may interfere with absorption of the fat soluble vitamins. Water soluble vitamin deficiencies are most commonly caused by alcoholism (most of the B vitamins are inactivated by alcohol).

Vitamin A

In 1912, two groups of scientists working independently discovered that there was a substance contained in butterfat that was vital to the growth of animals. Laboratory animals would grow at normal rates for up to 4 months, but at that time all growth would stop, unless they received the compound. In 1930 the substance was identified as vitamin A. Other work identified the existance of compounds that can be converted into vitamin A. Known as the carotenes, they are said to be precursors of vitamin A.

Functions. Vitamin A is probably involved in more bodily functions than any other vitamin. The most well known of these being maintenance of the visual purple in the eye. Visual purple is responsible for vision in reduced light, and a deficiency of vitamin A leads to the well known symptom of night blindness.

Vitamin A is intricately involved with growth, and as mentioned, this was the first function that was identified with it. Before isolation of the actual chemical structure of vitamin A, foods were rated for their vitamin A content by the amount of growth they would permit in laboratory animals.

Another function of vitamin A is maintenance of the epithelial tissues. Good healthy skin and mucous membranes are vitally dependent upon adequate vitamin A. Without adequate vitamin A, the skin becomes scaly and dry. Vitamin A is thought to possibly be involved in the immune response, but the role is not clearly understood. All that is really known is that deficiencies will increase infections, particularly respiratory infections. Whether vitamin A takes an active part in the immunity system, or whether the weakened epithelial tissues and mucous membranes (as found in the lung) are responsible, it isn't known.

Deficiency symptoms. Vitamin A deficiency is the most common vitamin deficiency in the world. Severe deficiencies occur with frequency among populations in underdeveloped countries who subsist on diets high in cereal grains or rice. In the industrialized countries, less severe deficiencies occur in individuals who consume diets low in vegetables and dairy products.

The first symptom is night blindness, which is followed by a drying up of the tear gland. This causes the surface of the eye to dry up, and eventually causes sloughing of the epithelial cells of the cornea. Ultimately the cornea may rupture, leaving it open to infection and blindness.

By the time the tear gland of the eye begins to dry up, the epithelial tissues of the body also begin to become dry (and scaly). The most serious conditions occur in the mucous membranes, particularly in the lungs. Possibly as a result, persons suffering vitamin A deficiencies are more susceptible to respiratory infections such as pneumonia and tuberculosis. Disturbances in the intestinal tract (diarrhea) have been linked to degeneration of the epithelial tissue inside the intestine.

Toxicity. Excessive doses of vitamin A can be quite toxic. Vitamin A is the only vitamin in which toxicities may occur in nature. The livers of certain animals concentrate vitamin A in such high quantities, that eating the livers can produce toxicities. The most publicized toxicities came when Arctic explorers died after eating polar bear liver, an extremely concentrated source of vitamin A. Any animal that must undergo several months of deprivation, (such as Arctic animals) should be suspected of carrying excessively high levels of vitamin A in the liver. In most situations, the only food products that most consumers may come into contact with (carrying excessive vitamin A) would be cod liver oil, or possibly shark liver. The livers of common food animals (cattle, pigs, chickens) carry a considerable amount, but should be simply considered a good rich source for supplementing the diet.

Most commonly, vitamin A toxicities occur from overzealous use of synthetic vitamin A supplements. As explained on p. 3, folklore has dubbed vitamin A a cure for acne, which has caused teenagers to take excessive levels.[66]

The first symptom of toxicity has been reported to be headache. Presumably, this is due to increased intracranial pressure. Other symptoms have been reported to include nausea, loss of hair, thickening of the eyelids, and an exudate from the tear glands. The most characteristic (and catastrophic) symptom is spontaneous fracture of the bones.

The toxic level is approximately ten times the recommended allowance. The important thing to remember is that vitamin capsules are available at several times the recommended allowance. Prior to 1978, the FDA did not allow tablets that contained more than 150% the recommended allowances. However, in 1978 the health food lobby was able to get Congress to restrict the power of the FDA, and capsules are now available for human use that contain levels of vitamin A that would be useful only for veterinary use in large animal species.

The Daily Recommended Allowance of vitamin A in adults is 3500-4000 IUs. The toxic level is approximately 10 times that amount, 40,000-50,000 IUs taken over a period of time. One time doses of 500,000 IUs have been reported to cause death.[67] High levels of carotene apparently cause no physical harm, although the skin will turn a yellow-orange color.

Food sources. The richest sources of vitamin A are liver, butter, eggs, and milk. Carotene which can be converted to vitamin A

in the body, is found in green, orange, and yellow fruits and vegetables. Synthetic vitamin A is often added to margarine. The
following list includes some foods high in vitamin A value.

TABLE 18-1. FOOD SOURCES OF VITAMIN A.

Food	Portion	Vitamin A Value International Units
Liver		
beef	3 oz.	45,400
pork	3 oz.	12,600
chicken	3 oz.	10,400
Sweet potato	1	9,000
Carrots	½ cup	8,000
Spinach	½ cup	7,300
Peach	1	1,200
Green beans	1 cup	700
Milk (fortified)	1 cup	500
(unfortified)	1 cup	310
Cheese	1 oz.	300
Eggs	1	260
Orange	1	260
Butter	1 pat	150

Vitamin D

Vitamin D is of extreme importance in the nutrition of children.
Without proper levels, the condition known as rickets will occur.
Until the discovery of vitamin D, rickets occurred with frequency
among children in the U.S. and northern Europe.

With the introduction of synthetic vitamin D, another concern
developed. Given at levels of only 5 times the recommended
amounts, vitamin D is toxic. Overzealous use of supplements
by parents can lead to clinical toxicities.

If adequate sunshine is available, vitamin D can be produced
within the body. The body is able to synthesize a compound that
can be converted into vitamin D. Known as 7-dehydrocholesterol,
when the ultraviolet rays of sunlight strike the skin, the compound
is converted to vitamin D.

Functions. Vitamin D is intimately involved with the absorption and metabolism of calcium and phosphorous. Without adequate vitamin D, calcium and phosphorous are poorly digested. More importantly, deposition of calcium and phosphorous in the bone tissue is highly dependent upon adequate vitamin D. Without adequate levels, the bone growth in children is reduced and distorted, and in adults the strength of the bone is reduced.

Deficiencies. In children, vitamin D deficiency results in rickets. Rickets, of course, is characterized by bowed legs and enlarged joints. The reason for the bowed legs is that proper calcification of the bone does not occur, and so it remains soft. As the child increases in weight, the force exerted on the long bones of the leg causes them to bend - thus the bowed legs. The knee joints appear enlarged because they do not harden, and the weight they must support causes them to flatten out.

In adults, vitamin D deficiency results in what is known as osteomalacia. Without vitamin D, the calcium and phosphorous content of the bones is allowed to deplete. This causes the thickness of the bones to decrease, which makes them more susceptible to breaking.

Toxicities. With supplemental vitamin D, the danger of toxicity is substantial. This is because the range between what is needed to prevent deficiency and what will cause toxicity is very narrow. The recommended allowance for vitamin D is set at 400 IUs; intakes of only 2,000 IUs can be toxic.

Toxicity is apparently due to excesses of calcium in the blood, known as hypercalcemia. Outward signs can be reduced growth, calcium deposits in the soft tissues, or kidney stones. Ultimately, excessive vitamin D can be a life threatening situation.

As with vitamin A, it should be pointed out that supplements are available that contain levels that far exceed any need for the compound.

Sources. The best natural source of vitamin D is sunlight. Liver, egg yolk, and dairy products are the best food sources, but the levels are variable. Because food sources are variable, vitamin D is almost universally added to milk. As mentioned previously, milk was chosen because it is the best source of calcium in the diet.

Vitamin E

There has probably been more speculation about vitamin E than any other dietary compound. Food faddists have credited vitamin E with being capable of restoring fertility, libido (sex drive), preventing heart attacks, and even reducing the effect of aging. As a result, supplemental vitamin E products have been purchased and used in massive amounts. Fortunately, vitamin E is apparently one of the least toxic of the vitamins.

As discussed in chapter 1, the mystical properties attributed to vitamin E probably began as extrapolations of the deficiency symptoms it would cure in laboratory animals. The types of deficiency symptoms expressed vary greatly in different animal species. As a result, vitamin E has apparently been reputed to cure just about every type of major ailment.

The fact of the matter is that in humans, deficiencies do not exist except when there is some type of digestive disorder that prevents the absorption of fats. (Or when infants are fed poor quality formulas.) When this happens, the symptoms are non-specific. The only visible symptom has been overall poor health or growth (in children). Laboratory analysis has shown a shortened life span for red blood cells, an indication of muscle wasting, and changes within the musculature of the small intestine.

Requirement. The requirement for vitamin E cannot be accurately set for the public in general. The reason is that the requirement for vitamin E varies with the amount of unsaturated fats in the diet. The greater the intake of unsaturated fats, the higher the vitamin E requirement. The reason has not been clearly explained, but is probably due to the fact that the type of fat deposited in the body is related to the type of fat eaten. Vitamin E is an antioxidant (retards spoiling or rancidity), and this property is no doubt related to the increased requirement in relation to the type of fat consumed. To simplify matters, the foods highest in vitamin E are the unsaturated fats. As a result, people who eat diets high in unsaturated fats typically get the additional vitamin E they need. Table 18-2 lists the highest food sources of vitamin E.

Toxicity. As mentioned previously, vitamin E is the least toxic of all the fat soluble vitamins. Even though the taking of massive doses of the compound is widespread, there have been very few reported toxicities. Still, the National Academy of Sciences advises caution due to the known toxicities associated with the other fat soluble vitamins. Fat soluble vitamins are stored in the body,

TABLE 18-2. FOOD SOURCES OF VITAMIN E.

Food	Serving Size	Vitamin E Content (alpha tocopherol) (milligrams)
Safflower oil	1 tablespoon	3.54
Corn oil	1 tablespoon	2.99
Soybean oil	1 tablespoon	2.04
Liver	3 oz.	.52
Banana	1	.32
Ground beef	3 oz.	.30
Chicken (white meat)	3 oz.	.30
Butter	1 tablespoon	.13
Whole wheat bread	1 slice	.11

and no one really knows what the long term effect of illogically high levels of vitamin E may be (since the taking of high levels actually only began about 15 years ago).

Vitamin K

In the early 1930's, Danish scientists discovered that a substance contained in fat was required for proper blood clotting. They named the substance vitamin K, for Koagulation factor.

There are two sources of vitamin K; naturally occurring vitamin K in foods, and vitamin K that is synthesized in the intestine. Humans do not synthesize vitamin K directly. Rather, bacteria in the intestine do the actual synthesis, and it is apparently absorbed into the body with the fats digested there.

Because the intestinal bacteria can synthesize vitamin K, the National Research Council has not set a recommended allowance. Instead it has set what is termed "Estimated Safe and Adequate Intakes". The minimum level is set at 70 micrograms, which is easily met by a typical Western diet. Green leafy vegetables are highest in vitamin K, with animal protein products supplying lesser amounts.

The symptom of vitamin K deficiency is reduced blood clotting time. Because of the ability of intestinal bacteria to synthesize the compound, deficiencies do not occur in healthy people. However, prolonged taking of antibiotics which kill off the intestinal bacteria, can induce deficiencies. Neomycin has been implicated in this regard.[5] Also, any ailment that impairs fat absorption (liver, gall bladder, etc.) can induce deficiencies.

Newborn infants are susceptible to vitamin K deficiencies since it takes a period of time before intestinal bacteria populations develop. For that reason, most infant formulas contain supplemental vitamin K. Breast fed infants should be given supplemental vitamin K. There are different forms of vitamin K, and one of them is potentially toxic. For that reason, it is best to leave specific supplementation advice up to a pediatrician.

THE WATER SOLUBLE VITAMINS

The water soluble vitamins include vitamin C, and the B vitamins. Unlike the fat soluble vitamins, the water soluble vitamins cannot be stored in the body in physiologically significant amounts. As a result, there is a daily need for these vitamins.

In most cases, excess water soluble vitamins are efficiently eliminated in the urine. As a result, excesses of the water soluble vitamins do not carry the same toxicity danger that is characteristic of the fat soluble vitamins. The only water soluble vitamins reported to have possible toxicities (in massive amounts) are vitamin C, and niacin.

Vitamin C

Vitamin C is somewhat of an exception to the water soluble vitamins in that a certain amount can be stored in the body. Healthy persons can store approximately a 30 to 45 day supply. After that time, if dietary vitamin C is not supplied, within another 30 to 60 days scurvy will begin to appear. The first recognizable symptoms are what are known as petichial hemorrhages. These are small reddish spots on the surface of the skin. The next recognizeable symptom is usually bleeding gums. Aching of the ankles and legs will accompany severe edema (swelling) at the joints. Ultimately, scurvy can be fatal. In times past, scurvy was indeed fatal - causing severe losses in ancient armies and navies. Oftentimes more men succumbed to scurvy than combat. In the late 1700's the British Navy discovered that the consumption of citrus fruits and green vegetables would prevent scurvy. By the turn of the century, citrus fruit became a required part of military rations. Even with this knowledge, scurvy still occurred up until relatively modern times. As late as 1912, a team of explorers in the Antarctic died due to scurvy.

At the present time, the need for vitamin C is well known, and scurvy usually only occurs in infants fed unsupplemented formulas. In breastfed babies, if the mother's intake is adequate, her milk will also be adequate.

Indeed, at the present time the concern among health professionals is more the effect of excessive vitamin C intake, rather than a deficiency. Vitamin C is reputed to cure a wide range of ailments, and as a result a significant part of the population is consuming an enormous amount of synthetic vitamin C.

Requirement. Within scientific circles there is controversy concerning the requirements of vitamin C. Essentially there are two different levels that are considered in this controversy.

Experimental work with penitentiary inmates has shown that 10 milligrams per day will prevent scurvy. However, 10 milligrams per day will not saturate the tissues and create what is known as a vitamin C "pool". That is, create reserves to be called upon whenever vitamin C is deficient in the diet. About 45-60 milligrams per day are required to create a reserve pool.

There is some indication that vitamin C is required for body processes other than the prevention of scurvy. It is known that vitamin C is required for proper wound healing, fat metabolism, and iron absorption. For that reason, the National Research Council has set the recommended allowance of vitamin C at 60 milligrams; a level that will afford tissue saturation.

Stress or temperature extremes are known to increase the requirement further. Studies with South African miners has shown heat stress may increase the daily requirement to as much as 200 to 250 mg./day.

Toxicity. Excess vitamin C is exchanged at the kidney relatively easy. When a large amount of vitamin C is consumed, the majority of it is washed out with the urine. This is apparently the reason that toxicities of vitamin C are rare.

The only known toxic symptom is digestive upset and diarrhea. Over a long enough period, however, there is a side effect that can have substantial medical consequences. High levels of vitamin C in the urine are converted to oxalic acid which apparently precipitates minerals and tends to cause kidney stones. Other studies have reported excess absorption of iron, and impaired ability of the white blood cells to fight bacterial infections.

Megavitamin therapy. As the reader is well aware, "If a little is good, then a whole lot more is better" is an unfortunate, but very common attitude of much of the public. While nutrition has no patent on this concept, the subject of vitamins has been a prime example.

In 1970, a popular book was published that claimed that massive doses of vitamin C were effective in the prevention and cure of the common cold. This caused the public to begin consuming enormous amounts of ascorbic acid, and also caused the scientific community to begin a number of investigations.

Most of the legitimate trials have shown either no difference or only very slight differences in the occurance and/or severity of colds among people taking massive doses of vitamin C. In reviewing the scientifically creditable trials, one health authority has reported that subjects taking extreme doses of vitamin C were shown to have .09 fewer colds, and that they had those colds .11 fewer days. Since the long term effect of taking massive levels is unknown, he concluded that the very slight benefit did not warrant the potential risk.[18]

Food sources and cooking losses. Fruits and vegetables, of course, are the primary source of vitamin C. Table 18-3 lists some of the better sources.

TABLE 18-3. FOOD SOURCES OF VITAMIN C.

Food	Portion	Vitamin C (milligrams)
Orange juice	1 cup	120
Cantelope	½ mellon	90
Grapefruit juice	1 cup	84
Orange	1	66
Broccoli	½ cup	53
Strawberries	½ cup	44
Grapefruit	½ grapefruit	44
Spinach	½ cup	40
Potato	1 med.	31
Tomato	1 med.	28
Liver (fried)	3 oz.	23
Cabbage	½ cup	21
Peas	½ cup	11
Apple	1	7

Vitamin C is denatured by heat, oxygen, and metals such as iron and copper. As a result, not all the vitamin C contained in foods at harvest time, is still available at the time of consumption. Prolonged cooking and exposure to air are particularly detrimental to vitamin C contents. Reportedly, the use of iron or copper cooking ware can reduce the amount of available vitamin C.

This is compensated by the fact that a balanced diet supplies more than the recommended allowance of vitamin C. If a vegetable is eaten with every meal, and at least some fruit is eaten during the day, the vitamin C requirement will be more than met.

THE B VITAMINS

Orginially, all the B vitamins were believed to be one factor. When it was discovered that there was more than just one compound, the succeeding vitamins became known as the B vitamin complex.

Thiamine

Thiamine was the first vitamin to be discovered. As explained on p. 49, its chemical composition was identified in 1911. Prior to that time, it had been found that a balanced diet would prevent the condition known as beriberi. Beriberi was endemic among Japanese sailors who ate diets based on white rice. When unpolished brown rice was eaten, or animal protein products were added to the diet, beriberi did not appear.

Deficiency symptoms. The first symptom of thiamine deficiency is reduced reflexes (the knee tap reflex). As the deficiency continues, walking becomes painful and results in a characteristic high stepping gait known to be associated with classical beriberi. Further advancement of the deficiency results in a general inco-ordination. Apparently this is due to the fact that thiamine is involved in nerve transmission.

Prolonged beriberi results in either emaciation of the legs, or edema of the legs. In either case, weakness in the legs is very apparent. Reportedly this is a serious problem in many Asian countries, and limits the ability of the populace to perform physical work.

Ultimately beriberi can result in enlargement of the heart. If deficiency continues, death can result. Death occurs much more quickly in children than adults.

American prisoners of war held in North Viet Nam were reported to have suffered from beriberi. Due to the enrichment of white flour and rice, and the liberal use of animal protein products, beriberi in the U.S. and other industrialized nations is rare. When it does occur, it is usually the result of alcoholism. Alcohol greatly reduces the absorption of most of the B vitamins.

Other factors that tend to induce thiamine deficiency are raw fish which contains an enzyme that destroys thiamine, and tea which contains a thiamine antagonist. Obviously, these factors would tend to antagonize the white rice diet of Asian countries, and are probably part of the reason beriberi is so common there.

Food sources and cooking losses. The very best food sources are brewers yeast and wheat germ. The next richest sources are pork, followed by enriched bread. Thiamine is very heat stable so cooking does not destroy it. However, since it is water soluble, much thiamine can be lost in cooking if the liquids are poured off. For that reason, vegetables should be cooked in a minimum of water, and meat gravies should be saved. Table 18-4 lists some of the richer sources.

TABLE 18-4. FOOD SOURCES OF THIAMINE (VIT. B_1).

Food	Portion	Thiamine (Vitamin B_1) (milligrams)
Brewers yeast	1 tablespoon	1.25
Pork	3 oz.	.78
Pecans	$\frac{1}{4}$ cup	.25
Orange juice	1 cup	.24
Rice (enriched)	1 cup	.23
Bread (enriched)	2 slices	.22
Peas	$\frac{1}{2}$ cup	.22
Liver	3 oz.	.22

Riboflavin

After the discovery of thiamine (vit. B_1) it was found that there was a second water soluble factor required for growth. Originally called vitamin B_2, it was later named riboflavin for the flavo enzyme it is involved with.

Unlike other vitamins, when riboflavin is deficient, a serious deficiency disease does not occur. The only clinical symptoms of a deficiency are crusting around the lips and corners of the mouth, and in men, a scrotal dermatitis. In children, a retardation of growth will occur.

Food sources and losses. The richest source of riboflavin is liver. However, in the American diet, dairy products supply the majority of riboflavin consumed. The next best sources are enriched bakery products.

Riboflavin is very heat stable, but is inactivated by light. The current use of paper milk cartons as apposed to clear plastic or glass containers is better for the preservation of riboflavin. Like the other B vitamins, riboflavin is water soluble, and therefore pouring off the cooking juices of foods will reduce the content of riboflavin (and other B vitamins).

TABLE 18-5. FOOD SOURCES OF RIBOFLAVIN.

Food	Portion	Riboflavin (milligrams)
Liver	3 oz.	3.56
Milk	1 cup	.40
Beef (hamburger)	3 oz. patty	.18
Egg	1 large	.15
Asparagus	½ cup	.13
Cheese	1 oz.	.11
Broccoli	½ cup	.11
Bread	1 slice	.07

Niacin

A deficiency of the B vitamin niacin, produces a serious deficiency disease known as pellagra. The symptoms of pellagra are a severe dermatitis that results in a scaly redness and extreme itching and burning sensation. Further progression affects the mucous glands of the digestive tract which results in abdominal pain, loss of appetite, and diarrhea. As the deficiency continues, mental faculties are affected. Ultimately, the unfortunate individual may become demented. Paralysis and death can follow.

Pellagra used to be an endemic problem in the U.S. (see p. 49). At the present time, pellagra is a problem in African nations where the populace is forced to live on a corn based diet.

Relationship with the amino acid tryptophane. Research has shown that the body can synthesize niacin from the amino acid tryptophane. Therefore, foods such as dairy products that are high in tryptophane, but low in niacin are valuable anti-pellagra food sources. Conversely, diets that contain poor quality protein sources (vegetable proteins are low in tryptophane) are often typified by pellagra.

Food sources and stability. The best sources of niacin are liver, and muscle meats. Certain legumes, such as peanuts are also good sources. As mentioned, dairy products are low in niacin, but quite high in tryptophane, which makes them valuable in the diet. Fruits and vegetables contain low to moderate levels of niacin.

TABLE 18-6. NIACIN CONTENT OF FOODS.

Food	Portion	Total Niacin (including tryptophane) (milligrams)
Liver	3 oz.	17.0
Chicken	3 oz.	10.3
Beef	3 oz.	7.2
Peanuts	1 oz.	6.0
Milk	1 cup	2.2
Cheese	1 oz.	1.6
Egg	1 large	1.5
Corn (whole)	½ cup	1.35
Bread (enriched)	1 slice	1.2

Niacin is very stable to both heat and light. The only loss that may be anticipated with cooking would be the losses associated with cooking liquids (being water soluble).

Vitamin B$_6$

Vitamin B6 represents three different compounds which are

collectively known as pyroxidine. Apparently all three of the compounds are interchangeable in the body.

Unlike the other B vitamins, vitamin B_6 is not involved in energy metabolism. Vitamin B_6 is intimately involved with protein and fat metabolism. There is evidence to indicate that B_6 requirements increase when a high protein diet is consumed.

When B_6 deficiencies occur, there are no physical symptoms in adults. Infants may go into convulsions. In adults, the only signs may be depression and confusion. Biochemical experiments have shown reduced antibody production, which could be assumed to result in reduced resistance to disease.

Food sources. As with most of the other B vitamins, the best sources of B_6 are liver, and muscle meats. However, most foods contain at least some B_6.

TABLE 18-7. FOOD SOURCES OF VITAMIN B_6.

Food	Portion	Vitamin B_6 (micrograms)
Liver	3 oz.	840
Bananas	1	510
Beef	3 oz.	430
Cabbage	1 cup	160
Spinach	1 cup	150
Egg	1 large	110
Milk	1 cup	40

Vitamin B_{12}

Vitamin B_{12}, discovered in 1948, was the last vitamin to be identified. Prior to that time, it was known that consumption of liver would cure the condition known as pernicious anemia. Vitamin B_{12} was ultimately identified as the anti-pernicious anemia factor.

Ultimately it was learned that the human digestive tract contained a specific factor required for the absorption of Vitamin B_{12}. Known as the intrinsic factor, it was found that some people were incapable of synthesizing the compound. When this happened, pernicious anemia was the result. However, feeding levels many times the requirement allowed enough B_{12} to be absorbed to cure the ailment. Without this treatment, death was inevitable.

For normal people in the developed countries, vitamin B_{12} deficiencies do not occur. The recommended allowance is about 3 micrograms/day, but most Western diets supply at least twice that amount.

When B_{12} deficiencies do occur, it is typically in vegetarians, as plants are deviod of vit. B_{12}. Only animal protein products contain B_{12}. Table 18-8 lists the B_{12} content of some common foods.

TABLE 18-8. VITAMIN B_{12} CONTENTS OF SOME COMMON FOODS.

Food	Portion	Vitamin B_{12} (micrograms)
Liver	3 oz.	68.1
Beef	3 oz.	1.9
Fish	3 oz.	1.1
Egg	1 large	1.0
Milk	1 cup	1.0
Pork	3 oz.	.6
Chicken	3 oz.	.4
Cheese	1 oz.	.3

Folic Acid

A deficiency of folic acid will result in an anemia very similar to a vitamin B_{12} deficiency. Indeed, the two compounds appear to be interrelated.

In the developed countries, folacin deficiencies typically occur as a result of alcoholism. In the underdeveloped nations, folic acid deficiencies are a problem, particularly among pregnant women.

The food sources of folacin are liver, muscle meats, and green leafy vegetables such as lettuce and spinach. Diets high in cereal grains are typically deficient, and as a result, folacin deficiencies occur in less fortunate peoples.

Biotin

The B vitamin biotin was discovered when it was found that animals fed uncooked egg white developed a deficiency disease.

It was later discovered that a substance in egg white, known as avidin, makes biotin unavailable.

Experimental studies with humans revealed deficiency symptoms that include scaly skin, weariness, insomnia, depression, and generalized muscular pain. In one recorded instance, a naturally occurring case occurred in a woman who was consuming 6 raw eggs a day.

Biotin deficiencies do not ordinarily occur because biotin is widely distributed in foods, and is apparently synthesized by intestinal bacteria. Because biotin can be synthesized, a recommended allowance has not been set. The National Research Council has set a recommended safe level, which is approximately what is believed to be the average U.S. intake.

Pantothenic Acid

The name pantothenic acid is derived from Greek and is literally translated as "from everywhere". The implication being that pantothenic acid is found in nearly all foods. As a result, deficiencies of pantothenic acid are extremely rare. When they do occur, it is usually as a result of general malnutrition, and will occur alongside other B vitamin deficiencies.

To produce an uncomplicated pantothenic acid deficiency requires the use of a purified diet. Symptoms vary greatly with the species. The first investigations into induced deficiencies produced grey hair in rats. This prompted substantial speculation in humans, and folklore had it that supplemental pantothenic acid would prevent grey hair. Research into deficiency symptoms of pantothenic acid in humans proved this not to be true.

Actually, deficiencies in humans have relatively non-specific symptoms. Experimentally produced pantothenic acid deficiencies in volunteers resulted in insomnia, restlessness, and irritability. In children, symptoms would include poor growth. Severe effects in animals have been observed, and it would be reasonable to expect the same could occur in humans if deficiencies were allowed to continue. Again, it must be realized that experimentally purified diets are required to produce such deficiencies.

Recommended allowances have not been set. The National Research Council has estimated that 5 to 10 milligrams are adequate, and that intake in the U.S. varies from about 5 to 20 milligrams/day.

SUMMARY AND CONCLUSIONS

A well balanced diet will provide all vitamins in sufficient quantities. There is no scientific evidence that would indicate that massive levels of vitamins are beneficial. It is, of course, well known that massive levels of some of the fat soluble vitamins can produce toxicities. These effects are short term. What is not known at this time, are the possible long term effects of excessive but subtoxic levels of vitamin supplementation.

It is true that vitamin levels are often reduced during the processing and/or cooking of foods. In most cases, however, the amount of loss has been exaggerated. Where losses have been significant, they are often reversed through supplemental addition of synthetic vitamins. An example would be the addition of B vitamins to bakery products.

Probably the most significant losses occur among the water soluble vitamins. Being water soluble, the pouring off of cooking water or juices will often significantly reduce the vitamin content of food. For that reason it is usually best to cook vegetables in as little water as possible, and to save meat gravies.

Moreover, whenever vitamin deficiencies occur (in industrialized nations) it is usually the result of alcoholism, chronic metabolic diseases affecting digestion, or self induced malnutrition such as vegetarianism. Alcoholism often causes deficiencies by destroying several of the B vitamins. In severe alcoholism, the substitution of alcoholic beverages for nutritious foods obviously compounds the problem. Elderly people often have chronic gall bladder or liver problems which can interfere with fat digestion. Anything that interferes with fat digestion can interfere with absorption of the fat soluble vitamins. Vegetarians must take supplemental vitamin B_{12} as there are no vegetable sources of that vitamin.

If an individual is concerned about nutrition, it is far more beneficial to be concerned about a balanced diet, than taking vitamin supplements. Consumption of whole cereal grains instead of flour, sugar, or cornstarch, and adequate levels of fruits, vegetables, dairy products, and meats will ensure adequate vitamin intake. In addition, such a diet will ensure benefits of protection from a number of nutritionally related disorders, independent of vitamins. As explained on p. 55, if a vitamin supplement is still desired, it should be well balanced. Large doses of individual vitamins have no proven benefits, but many well documented detrimental effects.

Chapter 19   MINERALS

As the reader is well aware, minerals are required for normal functioning of the body. The amount of each mineral required depends upon its functions. Minerals involved in bone formation, or acid/base balance are needed in relatively large amounts and are known as the macrominerals. Minerals required only as comporets in enzyme systems are typically required in much lower amounts, and are known as the microminerals or trace elements.

When minerals are present in excessive amounts, a toxicity can result. The toxicity may be a result of the mineral itself, or a result of creating an imbalance with other minerals. The difference between the amount that is required for good health and that which will cause toxicity is often referred to as the requirement/toxicity range. In some minerals the range is quite wide; in others it is relatively narrow. Mineral toxicities have become a concern of health professionals, due to the current fad of ingesting high levels of minerals (and vitamins).

MACRO-MINERALS
Calcium

Calcium, of course, is a major constituent of bones and teeth. About 99% of all the body's calcium is in the bones and teeth. But calcium is also involved in nerve transfer and muscular contraction. Without adequate calcium, the body goes into a state of tetany, and death can result. To prevent this, calcium is mobilized out of the bones for use in the soft tissues. Mobilization is apparently greatest when dietary calcium is low. It has been estimated that on any given day, as much as 700 mg. of calcium moves in and out of the bones (the recommeded dietary amount is 800 mg. for adults).

When calcium continues to be mobilized out of the bones without replacement, the condition known as osteomalacia occurs. This is characterized by weakened bones, and is believed to be responsible for many bone fractures (breaks) in the elderly.

Calcium is contained in leafy vegetables, but the most important source in the human diet are dairy products. Without dairy products it is impossible to meet the recommended allowances. In addition to calcium itself, vitamin D is required for proper absorption. For this reason, vitamin D is routinely added to commercially processed milk.

Deficiency. The deficiency disease in children is the well known condition of rickets. (For a description, see p. 145.) In adults, osteomalacia would be considered the symptom. (see p. 145)

Toxicity. Calcium is relatively non-toxic, and it is virtually impossible to take in toxic levels with natural foods. However, through the use of calcium tablets or other supplements, it is possible to take in harmful levels. The only toxic symptoms of excess calcium are thought to be calcification of the soft tissues (calcium deposits), and possibly kidney stones.

Phosphorous

Phosphorous, like calcium, is a major constituent of the bones. Eighty-five percent of all phosphorous in the body is complexed with the bones. Phosphorous is also intimately involved in energy metabolism.

A deficiency of phosphorous would result in rickets (p. 145). As a practical matter, phosphorous deficiencies do not occur in humans. Even diets of poverty stricken people in underdeveloped countries typically contain enough phosphorous. Indeed, in the developed countries, there has been concern that the amount of phosphorous consumed may be excessive (in relation to calcium). In animals it is generally best to maintain at least a 1.5 :1 calcium: phosphorous ratio. In humans there is typically much more phosphorous consumed than calcium. The consequences of this are not known, but obviously are not severe. Probably the only thing one should conclude from this is reinforcement of the need for dairy products (the only practical natural source of calcium in the diet).

Magnesium

Magnesium, like calcium and phosphorous is a constituent of bones. It is also involved in nerve transmissions, and a wide range of enzyme systems.

Magnesium is widely distributed in foods. Leafy green vegetables, legumes, nuts, and meats are the best sources. This coupled with the fact that the kidney can regulate the magnesium level quite well, has made deficiencies a rarity. That is, when magnesium intake is low, magnesium is reabsorbed from the urine to maintain a proper blood level.

When magnesium deficiency does occur, it is typically as a result of alcoholism, general malnutrition, or kidney disorders. Experimentally produced magnesium deficiency has resulted in nausea and mental apathy. Further symptoms included muscular tremors and spasms.

Sodium

Sodium is what is known as an electrolyte. It has a number of functions, but its primary role is as a buffer. That is, it is used to keep the body from becoming too acid.

As the reader is probably well aware, the primary source of sodium is sodium chloride (table salt). Because of the widespread use of salt as a condiment in cooking and prepared foods, salt deficiency does not occur. Indeed, most people consume far more salt than they need. For a complete review of salt and salt toxicity (hypertension) see chap.8.

Potasium

Potassum is considered another one of the electolyte minerals. It has a role in maintaining the acid-base balance of the body. Potassium seems to play the dominant role inside the body cells, whereas sodium plays the major role outside of the cells.

There is some indication that a low potassium intake in relation to a high sodium (salt) intake may tend to aggravate hypertension. The fact that potassium is found inside the cells whereas sodium is found outside may have something to do with this.

Potassium deficiencies per say, do not ordinarily occur in healthy people consuming a balanced diet. For a potassium deficiency to occur, either malnutrition or some sort of digestive disturbance would have to occur (chronic vomiting or diarrhea).

Suboptimal potassium intake may occur in people substituting "junk food" for basic food staples. In this case, it should be pointed out that potassium supplements can be very dangerous. High levels of potassium can interfere with normal muscular contraction of the heart, and can therefore be fatal.

It is far better to simply consume natural foods high in potassium. Bananas and orange juice have long been considered two of the best. Other good sources include liver, meat, and legumes such as peas. Moreover, just a good balanced diet will supply all the potassum needed.

Chloride

Chloride is required by the body for use in electrolyte balance, and as a constituent of digestive secretions and cerebrospinal fluid. The most well known of the digestive secretions being hydrochloric acid, which is secreted in the stomach.

The primary source of chloride is common salt (sodium chloride), although other forms of chloride are contained in dairy products, and other foods. As a practical matter, chloride deficiencies do not occur in healthy persons. However, chronic vomiting or injudicious use of diuretics may lower chloride to the point of adversely affecting acid-base balance. In this situation, the form of reinstitution of chloride should be the decision of a physician.

TRACE MINERALS

Trace minerals, as the name implies, are required in very small amounts. In many cases, the amounts are so small that the actual requirement cannot be measured without using chemically purified diets.

As a general rule, trace minerals can be quite toxic when they are present in excessive levels. Toxicity can be due to direct action of the mineral, or through effect on other minerals. For example, high molybdenum ties up copper and makes it unavailable.

Iron

In the practical aspects of nutrition, iron is an extremely important trace element. Iron is required for hemoglobin synthesis and muscle growth, and therefore women and children have a higher requirement than men. Women, of course, have a higher requirement to replace blood losses during menstruation, and children have a higher requirement due to growth. During pregnancy, the iron requirement of women is approximately the same as that required to replace menstrual losses.

The National Research Council has concluded that it is difficult for premenapausal women to meet their iron requirements with the diet consumed by most women. Men can easily meet their requirement, unless they are habitual blood donors.

When calculating iron intake, one must not only consider the amount of iron in each food, but also other foods eaten simultaneously. Liver and meats are not only high in iron, but also increase the absorption of iron from other foods. It has been determined that the addition of animal protein to a meal, increases absorption of iron from vegetable sources 60 to 80%. In addition, foods containing vitamin C also stimulate iron absorption. Obviously then, well balanced meals are required for maximum iron absorption. Table 19-1 lists the iron content of various foods.

Deficiency. The ultimate symptom of iron deficiency is anemia.

TABLE 19-1. IRON CONTENT OF COMMON FOODS.

Food	Portion	Iron (milligrams)
Liver	3 oz.	7.3
Beef and pork	3 oz.	3.0
Spinach	½ cup	2.0
Peas	½ cup	1.6
Chicken	3 oz.	1.4
Potato	1 med. size	1.1
Egg	1	1.0
Bread (enriched)	1 slice	.7
Rasins	1½ tablespoons (1 pkg.)	.5
Orange	1	.5
Fish	3 oz.	.4

Iron is required to form hemoglobin which is the compound responsible for carrying oxygen in the blood. With a reduced amount of iron, the amount of oxygen the blood can carry is reduced. Physical work or exercise requires extra oxygen, and therefore reduced tolerance to work or exercise is the visible symptom of iron anemia.

Toxicity. It is usually impossible to get iron toxicity from eating foods high in iron. The one exception to that is in alcoholism, particularly when wine is the beverage used. Grapes are high in iron and alcohol tends to increase the absorption of iron. This has a particularly bad effect on the alcoholic, since liver damage is the main effect of excess iron toxicity.

While iron toxicity from foods does not ordinarily occur, toxicity from overuse of iron supplements occurs with frequency. The main problem is with children who ingest their mother's iron supplements. Approximately 2,000 cases of iron poisoning occur each year.[68] Iron toxicity can be fatal.

Zinc

The exact roles of zinc have not been completely defined,

but it is known to be involved in a number of enzyme systems. Zinc is important, in that the body is apparently able to store only relatively small amounts, and it is known that zinc is marginal in the diets of many people.

Liver and red meats are the best sources of zinc. Foods of vegetable origin not only contain less zinc, but the availability is much lower. As with iron, people who consume poorly balanced diets will be the ones with marginal to low intake.

The signs of low to marginal zinc have been reported to be poor wound healing, decreased or dulled sense of taste, loss of appetite, and in extreme cases, a form of dermatitis. Experimental work with animals has also shown reduced reproduction.

There have been no reported cases of zinc toxicity. Apparently zinc is much less toxic than other trace minerals. However, it has been reported that zinc excesses tend to tie up copper and thereby induce copper deficiencies. For that reason, it is best not to take supplements in excess of requirements. Moreover, the best advice is to simply eat a balanced diet. (High levels of zinc supplements have led to a mild toxicity which induced vomiting and gastrointestinal disorders.)

Iodine

Goiter (enlarged thyroid gland) is the clinical symptom of iodine deficiency. Goiter used to be a common problem in the central and western U.S., but the use of iodized salt has all but eliminated it. In other countries, goiter remains a problem.

Goiter is a problem wherever iodine levels in the soil are low. That is, food grown in a particular soil will reflect the level of iodine in that soil. For that reason, iodine levels cannot be given for various foods. Food levels are too variable.

In addition to goiter, a condition known as cretinism may occur in children born to iodine deficient mothers. Cretin children have protruding abdomens, enlarged tongues, and very coarse facial features. Mental retardation is often also a symptom.

In addition to goiter being caused by iodine deficiency, there are also compounds in various foods capable of preventing iodine absorption. Known as goitrogens, they have not been reported to have caused goiter in the U.S. Cabbage and turnips both contain goitrogenic compounds, and have caused goiter in animals fed high levels of these vegetables.

Toxicity. Iodine, a strong disinfectant, is obviously toxic, and is quite capable of causing death. In sublethal but excessive amounts it can cause a form of goiter. In northern Japan where seaweed is a part of the diet (seaweed is very high in iodine), about 10% of the population is affected with goiter.

In the U.S., bread is often treated with iodated dough conditioners, and there has been concern that some individuals may obtain an excessive amount of iodine. (One slice of bread treated in this manner would contain the entire daily recommended allowance.) However, there have been no reported problems.

Maganese

Manganese is a mineral known to be essential to animal species. Deficient diets produce poor reproduction, birth defects, retarded growth, and abnormal bone and cartilage formation. It is therefore assumed that manganese is essential to man, but there has never been a reported case of deficiency. Apparently the requirement for manganese in man is very low, and met by most diets. Whole cereal grains, vegetables, fruits and nuts are good sources of manganese, and would be included in the diets of most peoples.

Extremely high levels of manganese must be fed to animals to produce toxicity and apparently this is also true for man. Manganese inhaled as dust, however, is very toxic, and numerous problems with manganese miners and refinery workers have been reported. Manganese dust apparently works on the nervous system as impaired speech, and locomotion (walking) are symptoms reported to be characteristic.

Copper

Copper is known to be essential for animals. Inadequate amounts will result in a form of anemia, poor reproduction, and loss of hair pigment. Excessive amounts result in lethal toxicities.

In man, experimental diets have been unable to demonstrate a deficiency. Likewise, copper is apparently not nearly as toxic to man as it is lower forms of life. Because no one has been able to produce a deficiency in man, a recommended allowance has not been set. It has been estimated that ordinary intake would be 2 to 3 mg./day, and apparently that is quite satisfactory. It has also been estimated that intakes of up to 10 mg. would not cause toxicity.[5]

Fluorine

When laboratory animals are fed purified diets low in fluorine, reduced growth often results. It has therefore been assumed that fluorine is an essential mineral. However, because fluorine is contained in practically all soils and water supplies, a fluorine deficiency has never been reported.

The main interest in fluorine has come in its value in dental care. In the 1950's it was found that increased levels of fluorine in the drinking water could remarkably reduce dental cavities. At that time, a number of experiments were conducted, and it was found that increasing the fluorine content of water to afford an intake of about 1.5 mg./day, reduced dental cavities in children by over 50%.[5]

The exact action of fluorine is not clear, but it is believed the fluorine becomes complexed in the enamel of the teeth. It has been demonstrated that fluorine makes enamel more resistant to acid. It is therefore believed that this action makes teeth more resistant to the acid produced by bacteria in breaking down food remnants in the mouth, and therefore less susceptible to further bacterial decay.

It is also believed that fluorine becomes complexed in bone. During old age, calcium is known to flow out of the bone which weakens the bone and makes it more susceptible to fractures (breaks). At the present time, there is speculation that fluoridated water may be protective.

Toxicity. Fluorine toxicity is a problem with livestock grazed near bauxite mines and smelters. Bauxite (aluminum ore) is very high in fluorine, and severe toxicity problems have occurred with animals consuming contaminated plants or water.

In humans, serious toxicities are possible, but unlikely. There have been concerns about the danger of fluoridating water, but for a toxicity to occur, approximately 20 to 50 times the normal level of fluorine would have to be added and maintained over a period of years. Adding 2 to 5 times as much over a period of years, would simply result in yellow spots on the teeth, as is common in many areas of the U.S., where the ground water is naturally high in fluorine.

Molybdenum

Molybdenum is known to be essential to a number of animal species. It's essentiality could be proven only after laboratory techniques were developed to purify diets. Without such experimental diets, deficiencies cannot be produced. The requirement for molybdenum is exceedingly small, and all foods apparently contain adequate levels.

The primary concern about molybdenum in nutrition is its ability to tie up copper. High levels of molybdenum can induce copper deficiencies. Because of this, molybdenum should primarily be thought of as a toxic element.

Chromium

In the 1950's chromium was discovered to somehow be involved in insulin and glucose (blood sugar) metabolism. Since that time, sub-clinical deficiencies have been reported in humans. There has been speculation that chromium deficiencies may somehow be involved in diabetes, but there has never been any unequivocal proof of such a relationship.

As a practical matter, animal diets do not require chromium supplementation.[6] However, there is some concern that human diets may be marginal in chromium.[5] Presumably this is due to the amount of refined carbohydrate consumed by humans. Whole grains and unpolished rice are good sources of chromium, but when the bran is removed (in processing), so also is the chromium removed.

Supplementation with chromium would not appear to be wise. There is very little known about chromium, including the long range effects of toxicity. A far more prudent and practical approach would be consumption of a balanced diet. Substitution of whole grains and brown rice (as recommended in chapter 6 for weight control) for refined flour, sugar, cornstarch, and polished rice would substantially increase chromium in the diet. Meat and cheese are also good sources.

Selenium

Selenium is an essential element and is of prime interest because it has a very narrow range between deficiency and toxicity. In livestock, both natural deficiencies and toxicities frequently occur. In animal species it has been determined that the requirement is exceedingly small; only .1 part per million of the diet. Levels of 3 parts per million are toxic.

In man, neither deficiencies nor toxicities have been reported. However, because selenium is known to be highly toxic in animals, there is great concern about toxicity due to the recent availability of selenium supplements. Prior to the 1970's, it was illegal to sell selenium supplements, due to the potential toxicity. This placed a hardship on certain areas of animal agriculture, since selenium deficiencies are a problem in several geographic locations. The law was therefore changed and selenium supplements are now available for a number of species, including man.

Toxicity in animals results in lameness and sloughing of the hooves, loss of hair, cirrhosis of the liver, blindness, paralysis, heart atrophy, and death. In addition to immediate toxicity symptoms, extreme birth defects have been noted. Lack of eyes, feet, or wings in birds have been reported.

Most toxicities in animals are the result of what are known as accumulator plants. These are plants that tend to absorb an abnormal amount of selenium. Most of these are range plants, and man would therefore ordinarily not have contact with them.

The exact role selenium plays in the body has never been identified. It is believed that it plays a role in preventing oxidation of the cells, but other roles are certainly possible. It is also known that selenium has a close relationship with vitamin E, but again, the exact mechanisms have not been elucidated. In studies with animals, vitamin E can sometimes prevent deficiencies from occurring on selenium deficient diets. In some cases certain specific symptoms are prevented, whereas others are not.

Because of this relationship with vitamin E, there may be a certain amount of danger to the public. Health faddists have advocated taking high levels of vitamin E, for a variety of reasons. Fortunately, vitamin E is apparently one of the least toxic of all the vitamins and minerals. Selenium is not. If health faddists were to recommend selenium supplementation (because of its relationship with vit. E), a substantial danger would be created.

It should be remembered that no cases of deficiency in humans have ever been recorded. The requirement for selenium is exceedingly small, and a balanced diet provides adequate levels. Meat, milk, and whole cereal grains supply most of the selenium in the diet.

SUMMARY

With the possible exception of fluorine, and iron (for women), a well balanced diet will supply all minerals in sufficient quantities.

Many areas that are low in fluorine have fluoridated the water system. If you do not know the level of fluorine in your water, a local dentist would most likely be aware of what it is. If fluorine levels are low, fluorine can be administered in other ways. The most common being fluoridated tooth paste. Fluorine tablets are available, but before using them, the advice of a local dentist should be solicited. Taking too high a level will result in mottled brown spots on the teeth. (Very high levels, of course, can be toxic.)

The National Research Council has determined that it is difficult for premenapausal women to meet their iron requirement with the type of diet usually consumed. The main determining factor is the amount of meat consumed. Meat is not only high in iron, but increases absorption from vegetable sources. During pregnancy, most physicians will prescribe an iron supplement.

A well balanced diet will supply all other minerals in sufficient quantities. Imbalanced diets, will result in marginal quantities.

The most pronounced mineral deficiency will occur if adequate dairy products are not consumed. Dairy products supply 60 to 70% of all the calcium in the diet. An adult requires two glasses of milk or two ounces of cheese per day. In addition to calcium, milk is the only reliable source of vitamin D, which is required for proper calcium absorption.

Consuming inadequate amounts of meat or poultry may produce a marginal zinc deficiency. Chromium may also be at suboptimal levels if sufficient meat or poultry is not consumed. Likewise, the substitution of refined carbohydrates for whole cereal grains may result in suboptimal chromium.

The requirements for minerals are complex. Rather than utilize supplements, it is simpler to utilize a balanced diet. Balanced diets, of course, yield more benefits than just proper mineral nutrition. Unbalanced diets, with mineral supplementation, are far and away inferior for overall health.

Chapter 20 BASIC DIGESTION AND METABOLISM

ANATOMY AND PHYSIOLOGY OF DIGESTION

Figure 20-1 represents the organs in the human digestive tract. Most people recognize the stomach, and the small and large intestines as vital to digestion. However, the secretions from the pancreas, gall bladder, and liver are also vital to digestion. For example, without the bile secreted by the liver and gall bladder, the fat soluble vitamins (A, D, E, and K) could not be absorbed.

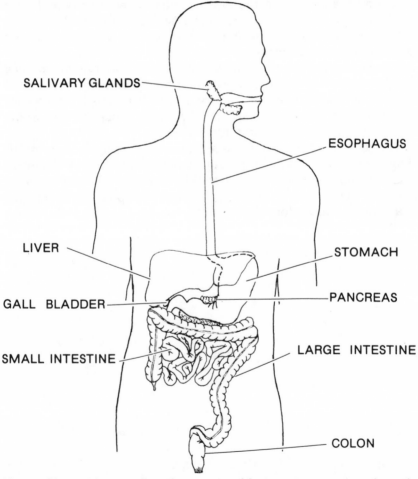

Figure 20-1. Human digestive tract. Most everyone recognizes the stomach and intestines as vital to digestion. However, the liver, gall bladder, and pancreas are also vital to proper digestion.

Digestion actually begins in the mouth, as the saliva mixed with the food contains a digestive enzyme. Saliva contains amylase, an enzyme used in the digestion of starch.

Once in the stomach, the food comes into contact with some extremely powerful digestive secretions. One of the most powerful being hydrochloric acid, which can liquify meat. The walls of the stomach are lined with mucus to protect them from the hydrochloric acid and other protein digesting enzymes. Without this mucous lining, the stomach would be digested by its own secretions. (This is why alcoholics often develop stomach ulcers - alcohol tends to dissolve away the mucous membrane of the stomach.)

The amount of time food stays in the stomach depends on the type of food. Carbohydrates leave the quickest. Fat stays the longest; up to 3½ hours. This is one reason meals containing fat have satiety value (prolong the return of the hunger sensation).

Upon leaving the stomach, the food is in a liquid form (chyme). It then enters the upper end of the small intestine, known as the duodenum. The duodenum secretes a buffer solution to neutralize the strong acid content that has come from the stomach. At approximately the same time, the gall bladder and the pancreas release digestive secretions into the duodenum.

The gall bladder secretes bile which is actually synthesized in the liver, but stored in the gall bladder. Bile is vital for proper fat digestion. The pancreas secretes another enzyme involved in fat digestion, known as pancreatic lipase. The purpose of these enzymes is to break down and emulsify the fat for absorption.

The pancreas also secretes a starch digesting enzyme, known as pancreatic amylase. Starch consists of thousands of individual glucose molecules bonded together, and pancreatic amylase breaks those bonds. The individual glucose units can then be absorbed for energy. In addition to amylase, there are also enzymes secreted which are specific for other types of carbohydrate. There is sucrase, for sucrose (table sugar), maltase for maltose (a sugar found in grains), lactase for lactose (milk sugar), and so on. An interesting but unexplained aspect of the enzyme lactase, is that non-caucasian races are often lacking the enzyme. As a result, these peoples cannot consume milk without suffering intestinal upsets. What happens is lactose escapes the small intestine undigested. When it reaches the large intestine, bacteria break down the lactose which results in flatulance (gas) and diarrhea. These peoples have the lactase enzyme during infancy, but apparently lose it during adulthood.

Absorption of most of the major nutrients occurs in the small intestine. Proteins, fats, carbohydrates, vitamins, and minerals are primarily absorbed from the small intestine.

What is left over from the small intestine enters the large intestine. The only nutrients absorbed in the large intestine are water and sodium. The large intestine is teeming with bacteria which often break down undigested foods. The method by which they digest foods is known as fermentation. A by-product of fermentation is carbon dioxide and methane gas. These are the gases that cause discomfort when certain foods are eaten.

At the end of the large intestine is the colon. The only nutrient absorbed in the colon is water. If much fiber is present, (which cannot be digested) a greater amount of water will be retained in the feces. This reduces abrasion to the colonic wall, and is apparently the reason diets very low in fiber have been linked with diverticulitis. The water holding ability of fiber also increases the rate of passage through the colon. Because of this, it is believed high fiber diets are protective of cancer of the colon. They reduce the exposure time that any carcinogen present in the feces can be in contact with the colon wall.

UTILIZATION OF CARBOHYDRATE

Carbohydrates are probably the most discussed, yet least understood constituent in the American diet. Most often, carbohydrates are lumped together as one entity. In reality, there are enormous differences between the different types of carbohydrates.

Basic structure. All carbohydrates are comprised of what are known as the simple sugars. The most common simple sugars are glucose and fructose. These simple sugars, known as saccarides, can be found in a free form, or bound together to form what are known as disaccarides or polysaccarides. A disaccaride consists of two simple sugars bound together, and a polysaccaride is more than two simple sugars bound together. The most common disaccaride is table sugar (sucrose), which consists of one molecule of glucose and one molecule of fructose. The most common type of polysaccaride is starch, which consists of long chains of glucose hooked together (Figure 22-2).

As mentioned, glucose and fructose can be found in a free (unbound) form. Fructose, often called fruit sugar, is the primary sugar found in fruit. Glucose is also found in fruits (and vegetables) but usually at lower levels than fructose.

In the small intestine, enzymes break compound carbohydrates into their constituent simple sugars. The simple sugars are then absorbed into the blood stream for use as energy.

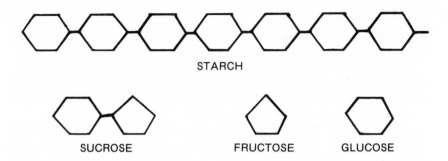

Figure 20-2. Chemical structure of starch and sucrose (table sugar).

Glucose metabolism. In order for glucose to be pulled out of the blood into body cells for use as energy, insulin is usually required. (During strenuous physical exercise glucose can be utilized without insulin.) The amount of insulin secreted depends upon the amount of glucose present in the blood stream.

When the blood glucose level is high, the pancreas will secrete a high level of insulin. That is, there is a set level of glucose that the body will allow to remain in the bloodstream. When this level is exceeded, enough insulin is secreted to remove enough glucose to bring the blood level down to the "normal" level.

If the body's cells need glucose for energy, glucose will be delivered to them for that purpose. When the cells no longer need any more energy, glucose will be converted into what is known as glycogen. Glycogen is simply a storage form of glucose. It is stored in the liver and muscles as a source of immediate reserve energy. When all the amount of glycogen that the body can store is met, the remaining glucose is transformed into fat, the other storage form of energy.

Fructose metabolism. Fructose is absorbed at a much lower rate than glucose. Fructose does not elicit an insulin response like glucose. In some cases fructose can be used as a source of energy directly, but the majority of fructose is converted to glucose (in the liver) before being utilized.

PROTEIN METABOLISM

Proteins are made up of what are known as amino acids. Different types of proteins will contain different amounts and sequences of the amino acids. However, there are nine amino acids that the body cannot synthesize. These amino acids are therefore called the essential amino acids.* Obviously then, proteins are essential for life. Indeed, the early Greeks were the first to coin the word protein, which means "before everything".

When protein containing foods reach the stomach, proteolytic enzymes begin breaking them down into their constituent amino acids. The amino acids are then absorbed into the bloodstream for possible use by cells in forming body proteins.**

If all the required amino acids are not present at the same time, body proteins cannot be formed. This is why "high quality proteins" (meat, milk, eggs, fish, and poultry), are so important in the diet. Vegetables, of course, contain proteins, but they are usually lacking in one or more of the essential amino acids. Grazing animals have specialized stomachs or cecums (a part of the large intestine) that contain microorganisms that can synthesize vegetable proteins into complete proteins for use by the animal. Simple stomached animals such as man, do not have such specialized digestive organs, and therefore must have all the essential amino acids in the diet*** (Figure 22-3).

Once the body's needs for tissue growth or replenishment are met, amino acids left over are used for energy. Excess amino acids are sent to the liver where they are converted for use as energy. The nitrogen contained in amino acids is removed, and excreted via the kidneys.

There are no reserves for amino acids. If enough protein is not eaten on a given day, the body will sacrifice protein from the muscles, for use in more vitally needed areas (blood cells, vital organs, etc.). This is why starvation type diets leave the dieter looking emaciated rather than just thin. Weight is lost from the musculature as well as fat stores.

*Histidine, isoleucine, leucine, lysine, methionine, phenylalanine, tryptophan, and valine are the essential amino acids.

**Inside each cell is what is known as DNA, which contains the amino acid code for that cell. Another compound known as RNA, retrieves and transfers the specific amino acids required for the construction of that particular protein.

***Vegetable proteins can be balanced to supply essential amino acids. For example, cereal grain protein is low in the amino acid lysine. Supplementing with soybean meal which is high in lysine does much to balance the amino acids. This is what is done in animal nutrition (for simple stomached animals). All ingredients of the diet are analyzed and a complete thoroughly mixed ration that contains all the needed amino acids is supplied. Theoretically possible in humans, as a practical matter, studies of vegetarian children have indicated subnormal growth.[70] This does not necessarily mean that vegetarian diets cannot be used successfully. Rather, what this probably means is that people do not stick to the rigid diet that is required for vegetarian diets to duplicate normal diets. That is, mixtures of vegetable protiens must be eaten at the same time, not separately.

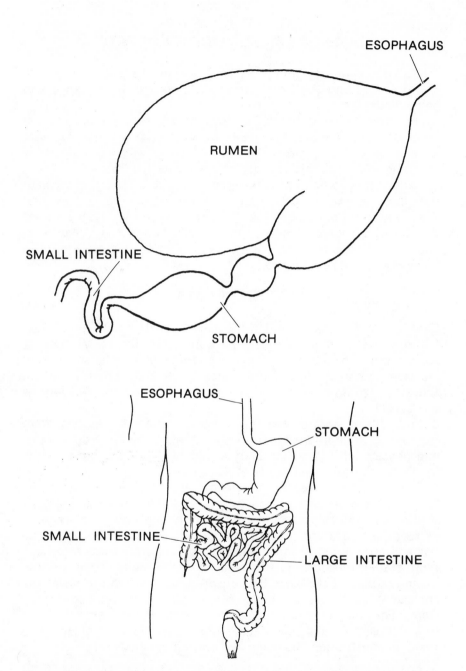

Figure 20-3. Digestive tract comparisons. Grazing animals have specialized stomachs known as rumens, which contain billions of microorganisms. These microorganisms are able to take incomplete vegetable proteins, and upgrade them into animal quality proteins.

DIGESTION AND UTILIZATION OF FATS

Fat digestion essentially takes place in the small intestine. The pancreas and the liver* secrete enzymes to break down and emulsify the fat.

In order for fat to be carried through the bloodstream it must be made water soluble. (By itself, of course, fat will not mix with water.) In order to make the fat molecules water soluble, they are complexed with carrier proteins, known as lipoproteins.

After fat is complexed with lipoproteins it is absorbed through the intestinal wall. Eventually the lipoprotein complexes find their way into the bloodstream.** From there they may be used directly as a source of energy in all cells except red blood cells, and nerve tissue (including the brain). Excess fats are stored in fat cells known as adipocytes.

TYPES OF FATS

Essential fatty acids. Through the use of purified diets it has been found that the fat linoleic acid is required by the body. Use of special purified diets result in a condition of rough, scaly skin. However, as a practical matter, nearly all diets provide several times the requirement for linoleic acid. As a result, deficiencies do not occur.

Saturated and unsaturated fats. For a variety of reasons there is currently great interest in unsaturated fats. The basic differences and physical effects on the body are known, but the mechanisms involved and the overall health effects are not.

The basic differences between saturated and unsaturated fats can be described several ways. As the reader is probably well aware, saturated fats are typically animal fats and are solid at room temperature. Unsaturated fats are typically vegetable oils and are liquid at room temperature. Saturated fats are much more stable; unsaturated fats become rancid much more quickly.

In the body it is known that unsaturated fats tend to lower the cholesterol content of the blood (see p. 101, for a detailed discussion). They also tend to increase the vitamin E requirement. Long term studies have shown that a diet high in unsaturated fats tends to result in unsaturated fats being laid down in the body fat.

---

*Liver bile is actually secreted from the gall bladder, a storage area for bile.

**Lipoproteins first enter the lymph system which later empties into the bloodstream.

Chemically the two differ in that unsaturated fats will have one or more double chemical bonds between carbons. That is, saturated fats look like this:

$$H-\underset{\underset{H}{|}}{\overset{\overset{H}{|}}{C}}-\underset{\underset{H}{|}}{\overset{\overset{H}{|}}{C}}-\underset{\underset{H}{|}}{\overset{\overset{H}{|}}{C}}-\underset{\underset{H}{|}}{\overset{\overset{H}{|}}{C}}-\underset{\underset{H}{|}}{\overset{\overset{H}{|}}{C}}-C\overset{\diagup OH}{\diagdown O}$$

Unsaturated fats will have two or more hydrogens missing, such as this illustration:

$$H-\underset{\underset{H}{|}}{\overset{\overset{H}{|}}{C}}-\underset{\underset{H}{|}}{\overset{\overset{H}{|}}{C}}=C-\underset{\underset{H}{|}}{C}=\overset{\overset{H}{|}}{C}-C\overset{\diagup OH}{\diagdown O}$$

Cholesterol. Cholesterol is not a fat, but it is a compound associated with the fatty portion of the diet. It is used as a base compound for a number of hormones, including the sex hormones. In addition to being a dietary constituent, cholesterol can be synthesized in the body. The amount synthesized in the body is usually related to the amount appearing in the diet. (For a complete discussion, see p. 94).

SUMMARY AND OVERVIEW

Protein, of course, is the vital ingredient in the diet. In order to meet bodily needs for amino acids, 3 to 4 ounces of high quality protein should be eaten at each meal. Proteins eaten in excess of that are broken down to form glucose. Glucose is required for use in the brain, other nerve cells, and red blood corpuscles. Most other body functions can use fats. If carbohydrate is absent from the diet, proteins will be broken down to supply the brain, nerve cells, and red blood corpuscles with the glucose they need.

Fad diets often presuppose that protein, carbohydrate, and fat metabolism are separate processes. In reality, they are intensely inter-related. The 3 primary hormones that control metabolism (insulin, adrenalin, and glucogan), all exert an effect on proteins, carbohydrates, and fats. There is therefore no real advantage to imbalancing the diet to afford weight loss. However, as discussed in chapter 5, there are some metabolic problems associated with eating imbalanced diets (as recommended by some of the fad diet plans).

REFERENCES CITED

1. R.E. Leakey. The Making of Mankind. 1981. Rainbird Publishing, London.
2. Victor Herbert. Will questionable nutrition overwhelm nutritional science. 1981. Am. Journal of Clinical Nutrition 34:2848.
3. Jean Mayer. Obesity. In: Modern Nutrition in Health and Disease. 1980. Lea & Febiger, Philadelphia.
4. Helen Andrews Guthrie. Introductory Nutrition. 1979. C.V. Mosby Co., St. Louis.
5. National Research Council. Recommended Dietary Allowances. 1980. National Academy of Sciences, Washington D.C.
6. Stephen Havas, and Sheila Pohl. Exercise and Your Heart. 1981. National Institute of Health Pub. #81-1677.
7. C. Martinez-Torres. Effects of cysteine on iron absorption in man. 1981. Am. Journal of Clinical Nutrition 34:322.
8. C.R. Myers. The Official YMCA Physical Fitness Handbook. 1975. Popular Library, Terre Haute, Indiana.
9. Bill Ryan. The government's suprising new position. 1981. Parade Magazine, Nov. 15.
10. Spencer Shaw and C.S. Lieber. Nutrition and Alcoholism. In: Modern Nutrition in Health and Disease. 1980. Lea & Febiger, Philadelphia.
11. E.D. Wison, K.H. Fisher, and P.A. Garcia. Principles of Nutrition. 1979. John Wiley & Sons, New York.
12. W. Koers, et. al. Preshipment feeding levels of calves. 1975. Amer. Journal of Animal Science 41:408.
13. D.N. McMurray, et. al. Development of impaired cell mediated immunity in mild and moderate malnutrition. 1981. Am. Journal of Clinical Nutrition 34:68.
14. A.E. Axelrod. Nutrition in Relation to Immunity. In: Modern Nutrition in Health and Disease. 1980. Lea & Febiger, Philadelphia.
15. M.J. Pertschick, et. al. Immunocompetency in anorexia nervosa. 1982. Am. Journal of Clincal Nutrition. 35:968.
16. W.R. Beisel, et. al. Single nutrient effects of immunogenic functions. 1981. Journal Am. Medical Assoc. 245:53.
17. D.J. Drutz, and J. Mills. Immunity and Infection. In: Basic & Clinical Immunology. 1980. Lange Medical Publications, Palo Alto.
18. R.E. Hodges. Ascorbic Acid. In: Modern Nutrition in Health and Disease. 1980. Lea & Febiger, Philadelphia.
19. H.H. Fudenberg, and J. Wybran. Experimental Immunotherapy. In: Basic & Clinical Immunology. Lange Medical Publications, Palo Alto.
20. Sharon Sobell. Helping the Hyperactive Child. 1978. Dept. Health, Educ. & Welfare Pub. #78-561.
21. P.L. Pipes. Nutrition in Infancy and Childhood. 1977. C.V. Mosby Co., St. Louis.
22. B.F. Feingold. Why Your Child Is Hyperactive. 1974. Random House, New York.
23. M.J. Sheridan and K.A. Meister. Food Additives and Hyperactivity. 1982. Amer. Council on Science and Health, New York.
24. B.F. Feingold and H.S. Feingold. The Feingold Cookbook for Hyperactive Children. 1979. Random House, New York.
25. E.H. Wender. Hyperactivity and the Food Additive Free Diet. In: Nutrition and Medical Practice. A.V.I. Publishing, Westport, New York.
26. N.N. Sharief and Ian MacDonald. Differences in dietary induced thermogenesis with various carbohydrates in normal and abnormal men. 1982. Am. Journal of Clinical Nutrition 35:267.
27. G.J. Friedman. Diet in the Treatment of Diabetes Mellitus. In: Modern Nutrition in Health and Disease. 1980. Lea & Febiger, Philadelphia.
28. Report of the National Commission on Diabetes to the Congress of the U.S.

1976. Dept. Health, Educ., & Welfare Pub. #76-1018.

29. John Yudkin. Dietary Intake of Carbohydrate in Relation to Diabetes and Atherosclerosis. In: Carbohydrate Metabolism and Its Disorders. 1968. Academic Press, New York.

30. Otto Schaefer, et. al. General and nutritional health in two Eskimo populations at different stages of acculturation. 1980. Canadian Journal of Public Health 71:219.

31. National Heart and Lung Institute Task Force on Arteriosclerosis. 1971. Dept. Health, Educ., & Welfare Pub. #72-219.

32. W.F. Ganong. Review of Medical Physiology. 1979. Lange Medical Publications, Palo Alto.

33. National Research Council. Toward Healthful Diets. 1980. National Academy of Sciences, Washington D.C.

34. A.C Marsh, et. al. The Sodium Content of Your Food. 1980. USDA Pub. #233.

35. R.M. Kark, and J.H. Oyama. Nutrition, Hypertension, and Kidney Disease. In: Modern Nutrition in Health and Disease. 1980. Lea & Febiger, Philadelphia.

36. Ruth Carol. Diet Modification: Can it reduce the risk of heart disease? 1981. Amer. Council on Science and Health, New York.

37. W.F. Enos, et. al. Coronary disease among U.S. soldiers killed in action in Korea: Preliminary report. 1953. Journal of the Amer. Medical Assoc. 152:1090.

38. J.J. McNamara, et. al. Coronary artery disease in combat casualties in Viet Nam. 1971. Journal of the Amer. Medical Assoc. 216:1185.

39. J.E. Rossouw, et. al. The effect of skim milk, yogurt, and full cream milk on human serum lipids. 1981. Amer. Journal of Clinical Nutrition 34:351.

40. S.W. Rabkin, et. al. Relationship of weight-loss and cigarette smoking to changes in high-density lipoprotein cholesterol. 1981. Amer. Journal of Clinical Nutrition 34:1764.

41. John Yudkin. Dietary factors in arteriosclerosis. 1978. Lipids, Vol. 13, No. 5:370.

42. E.J. Schaefer, et. al. The effects of low cholesterol, high polyunsaturated fat, and low fat diets on plasma lipid and lipoprotein cholesterol levels in normal and hypercholesterolemic subjects. 1981. Amer. Journal of Clinical Nutrition 34:1758.

43. G.M. Kostner, et. al. The influence of various diets on Type V hyperlipoproteinemia in children. In: Diet and Drugs in Atherosclerosis. 1980. Raven Press, New York.

44. L.H. Thomas, et. al. Hydrogenated oils and fats: the presence of chemically modified fatty acids in human adipose tissue. 1981. Amer. Journal of Clinical Nutrition 34:877.

45. G. Noseda, B. Lewis, and R. Paoletti. Diet and Drugs in Atherosclerosis. 1980. Raven Press, New York.

46. Otto Schaefer. When the Eskimo comes to town. 1971. Nutrition Today Vol. 6, no. 6.

47. R.E. Leakey. Origens. 1979. E.P Dutton Co., New York.

48. John Yudkin. Sugar and coronary disease. In: Controversy In Internal Medicine. 1974. W.B. Saunders Co., Philadelphia.

49. M. Sokolow and M.B. McIlroy. Clinical Cardiology. 1981. Lange Medical Publications, Palo Alto.

50. R.B. Chevalier, et. al. Reaction of nonsmokers to carbon monoxide inhalation. Cardiopulmonary responses at rest and during exercise. 1966. Journal of the Amer. Medical Assoc. 198:1061.

51. The health consequences of smoking. Report of the Surgeon General. 1971. Public Health Service, Washington, D.C.

52. AMA, Council on Scientific Affairs. AMA concepts of nutrition and health. 1979. Journal of the Amer. Medical Assoc. 242:2335.

53. Nancy Ernst, and R.I. Levy. Diet, Hyperlipidemia, and Atherosclerosis. In: Modern Nutrition in Health and Disease. 1980. Lea & Febiger, Philadelphia.

54. M.E. Shils. Nutrition and Neoplasia. In: Modern Nutrition in Health and Disease. 1980. Lea & Febiger, Philadelphia.

55. L.N. Kolonel, et. al. Association of diet and place of birth with stomach cancer incidence in Hawaiian Japanese and Caucasions. 1981. Amer. Journal of Clinical Nutrition 34:2478.

56. E.M. Whelan, et. al. Cancer in the U.S.: Is there an epidemic? 1981. Amer. Council on Science and Health, New York.

57. G.A. Spiller, and H.J. Freeman. Recent advances in dietary fiber and colorectal diseases. 1981. Amer. Journal of Clinical Nutrition 34:1145.

58. E.N. Alcantara, and E.W. Speckmann. Diet, nutrition, and cancer. In: Controversies in Clinical Nutrition. 1980. George F. Stickley Co., Philadelphia.

59. J.H. Hankin, et. al. Diet and breast cancer: a review. 1978. Amer. Journal of Clinical Nutrition 31:2005.

60. Otto Schaefer. The changing pattern of neoplastic disease in Canadian Eskimos. 1975. Canadian Medical Assoc. Journal 112:1399.

61. U.S. Dept. Health, Educ., and Welfare. 1980. National Institute of Health Pub. #80-2039.

62. H.R. Roberts. Food Additives. In: Food Safety. 1981. Wiley Interscience, New York.

63. American Cancer Society. 1982 Cancer Figures and Statistics. Amer. Can. Society, New York.

64. G.M. Gray, and M.R. Fogel. Nutritional Aspects of Dietary Carbohydrate. In: Modern Nutrition in Health and Disease. 1980. Lea & Febiger, Philadelphia.

65. Hugh Trowell. The development of the concept of dietary fiber in human nutrition. 1978. Amer. Journal of Clinical Nutrition 31:53.

66. Victor Herbert. Toxicity of 25,000 IU vitamin A supplements in "health" food users. 1982. Amer. Journal of Clinical Nutrition 35:185.

67. D.C. Church and W.G. Pond. Basic Animal Nutrition and Feeding. O&B Books, Corvallis, Ore.

68. National Research Council. Committee on Medical and Biological Effects of Environmental Pollutants. 1977. National Academy of Science, Washington D.C.

69. V.J. Liu and R.P. Abernathy. Chromium and insulin in young subjects with normal glucose tolerance. 1982. Amer. Journal of Clinical Nutrition 35:661.

70. J.T. Dwyer, et. al. Nutritional status of vegetarian children. 1982. Amer. Journal of Clinical Nutrition 35:204.

GLOSSARY

acidosis - see metabolic acidosis

adrenaline - The common name for epinepherine. A substance secreted by the adrenal glands during periods of strong emotion which results in a variety of effects upon the body. The most well known effects are a rapid increase in heartbeat and the metabolic rate. Simultaneously adrenaline causes a release of glycogen and fatty acids as an immediate source of energy.

aflatoxin - An extremely toxic substance produced by certain molds. Aflatoxin is believed to cause liver cancer.

amino acids - The building blocks of protein, comprised of an organic molecule connected to an amine group (NH2).

amines - Nitrogen containing compounds usually associated with amino acids. When found in their free form, amines are known to be capable of combining with nitrates to form nitrosamines, which are powerful carcinogens.

amylase - An enzyme used in the digestion of starch.

antibody - A substance formed in the body for neutralizing a specific invading organism or toxin.

antioxidant - A substance capable of reducing or eliminating rancidity in fats.

bile - A substance used in the digestion of fat.

bran - The outer coating of cereal grains, which contains most of the fiber and much of the vitamins and minerals. The bran is removed during the milling of white flour, corn starch, etc.

calorie - The amount of energy required to raise the temperature of 1 gram of water 1 degree centigrade. When used in reference to human food, it is kilocalories that is actually referred to. A kilocalorie is 1,000 small calories.

capillaries - The many tiny blood vessels near the surface of the skin.

carbohydrate - The type of energy produced in plants as the end product of photosynthesis (the process of turning solar energy into plant energy). The chemical structure of carbohydrates consists of carbon, hydrogen, and oxygen. (see also complex carbohydrates)

carcinogen- A substance known or believed to cause cancer.

cardiovascular system - The heart, lungs, blood, arteries, and veins. Everything required to deliver oxygen to the body tissues.

carotene - A compound contained in plants which the body can convert into vitamin A.

cholesterol - A compound synthesized by animals and used as the basic building block for a number of hormones and steroids.

complex carbohydrates - Usually refers to unrefined carbohydrates. That is, starch is usually surrounded by a fiber-protein complex which slows up the digestion of the starch contained within. Refined carbohydrates typically have this matrix removed, which makes them more concentrated, and quicker to digest.

dermatitis - Any condition which refers to rough, scaly skin.

diabetes mellitus - Inability of the body to regulate insulin, which results in abnormal glucose metabolism. Commonly called "sugar diabetes". The other common type of diabetes is known as diabetes insipidus, which involves abnormal secretion of vasopressin, the hormone involved in water regulation by the kidney.

duodenum - The part of the small intestine which connects to the stomach. Many enzymes are secreted into the duodenum.

electrolyte - An element such as calcium, potassium, chlorine, etc. which carries an electric charge. In the body, electrolytes perform a number of functions. Among them are regulation of the acidity of the blood, and passing electric currents along nerve junctions.

"empty calories" - Food items such as sugar and alcohol, which supply no nutrients other than calories.

emulsify - Commonly refers to the breaking down of fat into microscopic droplets for digestion.

enzyme - A chemical synthesized and secreted by living organisms for breaking down organic compounds.

epinepherine - see adrenaline

gall bladder - A small, greenish colored organ found attached to the liver which functions as a holding receptacle for bile.

germ - In cereal grains, the "embryo" portion of the grain (as in wheat germ), which is usually quite high in oil and vitamin E.

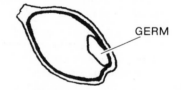

GERM

glucogan - An enzyme secreted by the pancreas which releases glycogen stores for use as energy.

glucose - A simple sugar commonly referred to as "blood sugar".

glycogen - The storage form of glucose.

glycoproteins - Proteins complexed with a carbohydrate.

goiter - Enlargement of the thyroid gland most commonly associated with a deficiency of iodine. (Large excesses of iodine can also produce goiter.)

hemoglobin - The compound in red blood cells required for the transport of oxygen in the blood. Iron is the central component of hemoglobin.

hyper - A prefix to many words which indicates an unnecessarily high level of something.

hypercholesterolemia - Unusually high level of cholesterol in the blood.

hyperlipemia - Abnormally high levels of cholesterol and/or triglycerides in the blood.

hypertension - High blood pressure.

hypo - A prefix which indicates a small or reduced level of something.

hypoglycemia - Unusually low blood glucose level.

immune response - The ability of the body to neutralize invading bacteria, virus, and other organisms.

immunology - The study of the ability of the body to ward off disease.

insulin - A compound secreted by the pancreas that is vital for proper carbohydrate and fat utilization.

interferon - A compound produced in body cells for protection against invading organisms.

isometrics - A form of exercise where one strains against an immovable object.

I.U. (international unit) - A form of measurement used to refer to the concentration of vitamins in foods or synthetic preparations.

ketones - Commonly referred to as ketone bodies. Organic acids produced during the oxidation of fats in the absence of carbohydrate.

ketosis - A pathological state which occurs when excessive levels of ketones build up in the blood.

Kwashiorkor - A metabolic disturbance caused by lack of balanced proteins in the diet. Results in a fat layer being deposited around the liver. The outward signs are a distended abdomen.

large intestine - The last major digestive organ in the body.

megavitamin therapy - A current health craze characterized by the taking of extraordinarily large doses of supplemental vitamins. Most commonly a folklore method of warding off disease, or the effects of aging.

menarch - The age at which young girls begin to menstruate.

metabolic acidosis - A condition whereby the blood becomes slightly acidic, which can result in coma and death.

monosaccaride - see saccaride

nitrate - The form of nitrogen absorbed by plants (NO_3). Nitrates can be harmful to health in several ways.

nitrite - a reduced form of nitrate (NO_2).

nitrosamine - A compound often formed when nitrates or nitrites encounter free amines in an acid environment (as would be found in the stomach). Nitrosamines are known to be a powerful carcinogen.

osteomalacia - Usually a disorder of the elderly, in which more calcium flows out of the bones than in, which greatly weakens the strength of the bones.

pancreas - A small organ found in the abdominal cavity which secretes a number of enzymes and hormones that are vital to proper digestion and metabolism.

placebo - A sugar pill. A valueless medical treatment often given to a "control" group in research (group not given the real treatment for comparison), or to hypochondriac patients.

polysaccaride - see saccaride

polyunsaturated fats - Technical definition means fats with 2 or more double bonds between carbons. Refers to most vegetable oils.

refined carbohydrate - see carbohydrate

rumen - The large paunch preceeding the true stomach in grazing animals which enables them to digest and utilize grass and forage as the sole constituent of the diet.

ruminant - Animal with a rumen - most grazing animals.

saccaride - Scientific name for a simple sugar. When two simple sugars are bound together, they are known as a disaccaride; more than two a polysaccaride.

saturated fat - Technical definition is a fat which contains no double bonds between carbons. Commonly refers to most aminal fats.

sessile - Something which is very inactive.

small intestine - The digestive organ the stomach empties into. Most of the nutrient absorption takes place in the small intestine.

sodium chloride - Common table salt (NaCl).

starch - A polysaccaride consisting of long chains of glucose (simple sugar) units hooked together.

stroke - A life threatening pathological situation in which a blood vessel in the brain becomes blocked, or ruptured - thereby keeping a portion of the brain from receiving oxygen and other nutrients.

sucrose - The scientific name for table sugar. Consists of one molecule of glucose and one molecule of fructose bound together.

triglycerides - A form of saturated fat most commonly synthesized in the body and utilized for energy.

unsaturated fats - Fats with at least one carbon to carbon double bond.

INDEX

additives (food)
    in cancer 76-77
    in hyperactivity 123-128

adrenaline 10, 11

aflatoxin 116

alcohol 65-67
    in cancer 130
    in dieting 41, 65
    in heart disease 106-107
    in physical stamina 65
    effects on vitamins 65, 112

amino acids
    as health foods 3-4
    requirement for 174

amines 22, 114

antibodies 71-72

antibiotics 69-71

atherosclerosis 94-112
    in diabetes 85
    risk factors 96

bacteria 69-70

beri beri 49, 151-152

biotin 156-157

bran 137-138

breast feeding (and cancer) .. 122-123

butter 40

calcium 53-54, 159-160

calorie 13

caloric values 13-18, 38

cancer (def.) 113
    breast 119-120, 122-123
    colon 116
    death rate 115, 118-119, 129
    liver 116-117, 127
    lung 128-131
    stomach 22, 114-116, 127

carbohydrate 172
    complex 15-17, 23, 27, 36, 39
    in diabetes 86
    in dieting 23, 27, 36
    refined 13-18, 27, 39

carbohydrate loading 31

cereals 41-42

chloride 161-162

cholesterol 97, 177
    and alcohol 67
    and atherosclerosis 94-102
    content in foods 97
    metabolism 98-99

cigarette smoking ... 107-108, 128-130

chromium 167

cirrhosis 67

cobalamin 155

colds (and flu) 72-73

copper 165

cooking (low calorie) 133-139

cottage cheese 35, 137

cured meats 115

Delaney Clause 123-124

DES 119, 126-127

desserts 29-30, 133-138

diabetes 83-87

dieting
    fads 22, 26
    pills 20, 26
    protein 23-24
    starvation 20-21

diverticulitis 132

drugs (used in livestock) 126-127

eggs 35, 40

empty calories 12, 27

estrogens 120-121

exercise 57-64
    and the heart 59-61
    and physical appearance ... 19
    as an aid to sleep 46
    caloric equivalents 34
    constipation 132
    persons who should consult
    a physician 61
    strength building 62-63
    value in weight loss 32-34

fats
    caloric value 26
    and cancer 116, 119-120
    general 176-177
    in dieting 24
    digestion (effect on vitamins) . 141
    metabolism 11
    removing from food 138, 139
    saturated & unsaturated . 176-177

fiber 132
    and cancer 116

fish 114, 115

fluorine 165-166

flu 72-73

folic acid 53, 156

fructose 173
fruit 28, 36
   and cancer 117-118
gall bladder 170, 171
glucogan 10, 11
glucose 9, 10, 11, 30-31
   metabolism 172-173
glycogen 9, 30-31
health food fraud 1-4
heart attacks 59
   and diabetes 85
   and hypertension 88, 89
high density lipoprotein 99
hormones 12
hunger 9-18, 30-32
hydrogenated vegetable oils .. 111
hyperactivity (in children) ... 76-82
   and food additives 76-77
   and sugar 78, 79-81
   and vitamins 78-79
hypercholesterolemia . 99-102, 109-112
hyperglycemia 84
hyperkinesis 76
hypertension 88-93
immunity system 71, 75
   in diabetics 85
infectious diseases 69-75
insulin 83
   and fructose 28
   and sugar 104
interferon 73-75
iodine.................. 54, 164-165
iron 48, 54, 162-163
   effect of alcohol 65
ketones 24
ketosis 24
kwashiorkor 116-117
lipoproteins (def.) 176
   and heart disease 99
liver
   storage of glycogen 9
low density lipoprotein 99
magnesium 160
manganese 165
meal skipping 21
megavitamin therapy .. 2-3, 46-47, 78-79, 149-150

menopause
   and heart disease 96
   and cancer 121
metabolic acidosis 24
minerals (general).....46-55, 159-169
   (see also individual minerals; e.g. calcium, phosphorous, etc.)
molds (in cancer) 116, 117
molybdenum 166-167
niacin................... 49, 153-154
nitrates 22, 114, 115
nitrite 118
nitrosamines 114, 118
obesity
   and cancer ....:.. 121-122
   diabetes 83, 86
organic fertilizers 47-47
osteomalacia 54
pancreas 170, 171
pantothenic acid 157
pellagra 49, 153-154
pesticides 125-126
phosphorous 160
physical attractiveness 19-21
pneumonia 69, 70
potassium 3, 161
primitive societies
   and cancer 120, 121
   and diabetes 84
   and heart disease 102
   and hypertension ` 90
protein 21, 23-24
   animal proteins 48
   in cancer 116
   in relation to fat 35
   metabolism 173-174
   requirement 34-35
   utilization by diabetics ... 85
pyroxidine 155
riboflavin 152-153
rice
   brown rice 37
rickets 48, 145, 159-160
salad dressing 36, 41
salt 88, 90-93
salicylates 76-77
sausage 35, 40
scurvy 49, 148-149

selenium 167-168
sleep 44-45
sodium.................. 90-91, 161
sour cream 40, 136
starch 15, 28, 172
stress
    emotional 58, 88
    heat 66
    cold 66
sucrose 172-173
sugar 27-30, 33, 34, 41-43, 44
    and atherosclerosis 102-106
    chemical structures 172-173
    in cooking 133-138
    and diabetes 84
tobacco 128-131
trace minerals (general) 162
triglycerides
    and alcohol 67
    in diabetes 85
    and sugar 104
ulcers 66
vaccination 71-72
vegetables
    in cancer 114-115
    in meals 35
    nitrates 22-23
vegetable fat
    and cancer 119-120
virus 69-71
    in diabetes 83, 87
vitamins 46-55, 141-158
    A 2-3, 50, 141-144
    B1 .... 49, 151
    B6 154-155
    B12............ 25, 50, 155-156
    biotin 156-157
    C 148-151
    C and stomach cancer . 22-23, 117-118
    content of food 47-49
    D 49, 52, 144, 145
    E 1-2, 146
    Fat soluble 141
    folacin 53, 156
    and infectious diseases .. 72, 73
    K 25, 147-148
    requirements 51, 56
    misinformation 1-3
    niacin 49, 153-154
    pantothenic acid 157
    recommended allowances . 50, 51, 65
    riboflavin 152-153
    thiamine 49, 151
    toxicities (general) 2-3, 141
    water soluble 141
weight loss
    recommended rate 26
whole wheat flour 137-138
yogurt 41, 136-137
zinc 163-164